PRINCIPLES OF DRUG INFORMATION SERVICES

A syllabus
of systematic concepts

Arthur S. Watanabe, Pharm.D.
Christopher S. Conner, Pharm.D.

PRINCIPLES OF DRUG INFORMATION SERVICES

A syllabus of systematic concepts

Arthur S. Watanabe, Pharm.D.

Rocky Mountain Drug Consultation Center
Rocky Mountain Poison Center
Denver Department of Health and Hospitals
Assistant Professor of Medicine and Clinical Pharmacy
University of Colorado Medical Center, Denver

Christopher S. Conner, Pharm.D.

Rocky Mountain Drug Consultation Center
Rocky Mountain Poison Center
Denver Department of Health and Hospitals
Assistant Professor of Medicine and Clinical Pharmacy
University of Colorado Medical Center, Denver

DRUG INTELLIGENCE PUBLICATIONS, INC., HAMILTON, ILLINOIS 62341

LIBRARY OF CONGRESS CATALOG NUMBER 78-50219
ISBN 0-914768-31-X

Printed in the United States of America by

THE HAMILTON PRESS, INC., HAMILTON, ILLINOIS 62341

CONTENTS

Preface

How to Use This Syllabus

The purpose of this syllabus is to provide the student with a means for the development and self evaluation of the skills required to function as a drug information consultant. The organization of this syllabus is based on the systematic approach, which is discussed and outlined in Chapter One. To obtain maximum benefit from this program, each chapter should be taken in sequence, since each chapter's information builds on that of the previous chapters.

The examples presented are intended to simulate some of the situations that may be encountered during student clerkship experience and practice following graduation into the "real world", and to provide a basic foundation on which the student can build his/her future experiences. This syllabus provides "self evaluation questions (SEQ)" for the student to assess his/her grasp of the main concepts stressed by the "Behavioral Objectives" and covered by the "General Discussions" sections. In addition, mock drug information questions are provided under "Learning Examples" to provide a mechanism for the application and practice of the syllabus' concepts. The learning examples are chosen to represent some of the most common types of questions that may be encountered and are not necessarily all inclusive. The student should note that learning processes are enhanced by active participation in the completion of these exercises, as well as by the application of these principles to his/her own experiences. It will be helpful to use this syllabus in an environment where reference and text sources are readily available, such as a medical library.

Special appreciation and thanks go to Drs. William D. Ball, David C. Bradford and James E. Knoben for their review of portions of this manuscript, and to the students of the University of Utah College of Pharmacy, Idaho State University College of Pharmacy, and the University of Colorado School of Pharmacy who demonstrated the principles of this syllabus to be practical.

Denver, Colorado 1978 Arthur S. Watanabe

PRINCIPLES OF DRUG INFORMATION SERVICES

A syllabus
of systematic concepts

1

Introduction to
Drug Information Concepts

Behavioral Objectives For Chapter One
Introduction to Drug Information Concepts

OBJECTIVE	CRITERIA FOR MEETING OBJECTIVE	SELF EVALUATION QUESTION NUMBER
The student should be able to:		
1.1 Demonstrate a knowledge and awareness of the functions of drug information services	1.1.2 Describe the role of the pharmacist as a drug information specialist	1.1
1.2 Demonstrate a knowledge and awareness of drug information services within the institutional setting	1.2.1 Describe the rationale and history behind the development of drug information services	1.1
	1.2.2 List usual services and functions of drug information services	1.2
1.3 Demonstrate a knowledge and awareness of drug information services that can be performed outside the institutional setting	1.3.1 Identify the services and functions of the pharmacist as a provider of poison and drug information in a community pharmacy	1.3
1.4 Demonstrate an ability to approach the answering of drug information requests using a systematic approach	1.4.1 Describe the systematic approach to drug information requests	1.4 1.5

The Role of the Pharmacist as a Drug Information Specialist

In 1966, Francke wrote in an editorial that the role of the pharmacist as a drug information specialist was essentially unfilled (Francke, 1966). Today there are over 90 functioning drug information services employing approximately two hundred full and part-time pharmacists (Rosenberg et al., 1976) and for all intents and purposes the drug information service is considered by the profession to be an integral part of pharmacy practice. However, despite more than a decade of experience since the first recognition of the pharmacist as a potential drug information specialist (Burkholder, 1963), can the pharmacist be said to be established in this role? Certain aspects of the literature shed some light on this problem. Studies, polling the attitudes of physicians, found that in the majority of cases physicians considered pharmacists to be a poor source of drug information (Zellmer, 1974; Moser, 1974; Smith et al., 1975; Harelik et al., 1975). Interestingly, these studies also determined that physicians considered the PDR and drug manufacturer detailman to be good drug information sources and relied on them more frequently than on pharmacists. To confound the situation further, Pearson questioned his own colleagues as to the necessity of the drug information specialist (Pearson, 1975) and suggested that the supply of such specialists was minimal, while a study by Halbert et al. surveying the 90 published drug information centers reported findings which further indicate that pharmacists "fall short in attaining their full potential for producing rapid, accurate and concise information about drugs" (Halbert et al., 1977). Discouraging as these findings may appear, it was also noted that physicians indicated that a drug information specialist could meet their needs better and that they were generally aware that drug information sources were lacking or inadequate. In addition, the Millis Commission report re-emphasized the importance of the pharmacist fulfilling this role. Thus, after more than ten years Francke's words still appear to hold true in some people's view; that is, the pharmacist has not yet fulfilled his/her calling as a drug information specialist.

What are the implications of these findings for pharmacists currently practicing as drug information specialists and those aspiring individuals training in the numerous colleges and schools of pharmacy? Ultimately, each individual must answer this question in a manner consistent with his or her own professional goals. However, two points are worth some thought. First, the studies mentioned previously indicate only where physicians would normally refer to for drug information and do not necessarily reflect on the ability or capability of the competent pharmacist to provide such information. In fact, these data may indicate a need to promote activities directed towards educating physicians on the benefits of utilizing clinically trained pharmacists for drug information (Leach, 1978). Secondly, Francke has also written that when social changes occur in a profession, they do not alter the attitude and values of its members until a significant number of members assume new roles and perform successfully in these roles for two or three generations (Francke, 1972). Thus it appears that it will require considerable time for the pharmacy profession to transform itself and to change its pattern of practice.

Then what is the status of the role of the pharmacist as a drug information specialist? At present, in view of the still unfilled need, it appears that pharmacists should continue to strive for the fulfillment of this role. The American Society of Hospital Pharmacists has published an official statement on the pharmacists' role in providing drug information services. This serves as a useful guideline or goal (*Am. J. Hosp. Pharm.*, 1968). In addition, Hirschman et al., in a monthly column entitled "DIAS Rounds", provided an exemplary "role model on paper" (Hirschman et al., 1970–72). Their columns emphasized the application of a philosophical approach to practical situations that has also been formalized elsewhere (Watanabe et al., 1975). The role they outlined utilizes the experiences and knowledge of the pharmacist, together with his ability to analyze and interpret drug information, to form the basis of professional services. In Hirschman's view, these consultative services should be designed to meet the needs of practitioners who present a drug or therapeutic problem concerning a specific patient (Hirschman and Maudlin, 1970). The reader is referred to these columns in the absence of a "live" role model.

Background Reading

1. Anon.: The Hospital Pharmacist and Drug Information Services, *Am. J. Hosp. Pharm.* 25:381–382, 1968

2. Burkholder, D.F.: Some Experiences in the Establishment and Operation of a Drug Information Center, *Am. J. Hosp. Pharm.* 20:507–513, 1963

3. Francke, D.E.: Development of a Professional Self-Image, *Drug. Intell. Clin. Pharm.* 6:49, 1972

4. Francke, D.E.: The Role of the Pharmacist as a Drug Information Specialist, *Am. J. Hosp. Pharm. 23*:49, 1966

5. Halbert, M.R. et al.: Drug Information Centers: Lack of Generic Equivalence, *Drug Intell. Clin. Pharm. 11*:728-735 (Dec.) 1977

6. Harelik, J.H. et al.: Pharmacist and Physician Evaluation of Drug Information Sources, *Am. J. Hosp. Pharm. 32*:594-597, 1975

7. Hirschman, J.L. and Maudlin, R.K.: The DIAS Rounds, *Drug Intell. Clin. Pharm. 4*:10-12, 1970

8. Hirschman, J.L. and Maudlin, R.K.: The DIAS Rounds, *Drug Intell. Clin. Pharm. 4*:45-48, 1970

9. Leach, F.N.: The Regional Drug Information Service: A Factor in Health Care? *Br. Med. J.1*:766-768, 1978

10. Millis, J.S.: Looking Ahead—The Report of the Study Commission on Pharmacy, *Am. J. Hosp. Pharm. 33*:134-138, 1976

11. Moser, R.H.: The Continuing Search: FDA Drug Information Survey, *J. Am. Med. Assoc. 229*:1336-1338, 1974

12. Pearson, R.E.: Drug Information Specialists—An Endangered Species? *Am. J. Hosp. Pharm. 32*:783, 1975

13. Rosenberg, J.M. et al.: Pharmacist-manned Drug Information Centers are Increasing, *Pharm. Times 43*:66-72 (Jan.) 1976; 42:56-64 (Feb.) 1976

14. Smith, G.H. et al.: Physician Attitudes Toward Drug Information Resources, *Am. J. Hosp. Pharm. 32*:19-25, 1975

15. The American Association of Colleges of Pharmacy: *Pharmacists for the Future: The Report of the Study Commission on Pharmacy,* Health Administration Press, Ann Arbor, 1975

16. Watanabe, A.S. et al.: A Systematic Approach to Drug Information Requests, *Am. J. Hosp. Pharm. 32*:1282-1285, 1975

17. Zellmer, W.A.: The Pharmacist as a Source of Drug Information, *Am. J. Hosp. Pharm. 31*:725, 1974

An Overview of Drug Information Services

As a result of increasing research, the identification and marketing of new drugs, changes in federal drug legislation and changes in medical and pharmaceutical care, there has been a significant increase over the past four decades in the volume of medical and pharmaceutical literature. From this "information explosion" has arisen the complex problem of communicating the latest information on drugs and their use to the health care practitioner. One solution to this problem has been the development of the clinically trained pharmacist as a source of drug information. Traditionally, pharmacists in both community and hospital settings have provided information to the health care professional by means of informal drug information activities. However, it was not until 1962 at the University of Kentucky that these drug information activities were formalized into an actual service by the organization and centralization of available information sources and the utilization of experienced and well-qualified personnel to disseminate more sophisticated drug information (Burkholder, 1963). It is the purpose of this section to define and describe drug information services.

Using a broad definition, "Drug Information Services" encompasses the activities of specially trained individuals (i.e., clinical pharmacists) to provide accurate, unbiased, factual information or consultations which are primarily given in response to patient-oriented drug problems received from pharmacists, nurses, physicians, and other health professionals. These services need not be limited to formalized "Drug Information Services" as they have been traditionally. Even an appropriately staffed and equipped community pharmacy can and should provide drug information.

Objectives

The objectives of providing drug information may include any or all of the following.

Service. The primary emphasis is on the effective communication of information arising from questions about the use of drugs in the patient care setting. This includes attempting to find documentation, in the form of articles or citations from the scientific and professional literature and, where appropriate, supplying advice such as the correct dosage regimen or dosage adjustments, potential adverse reactions or interactions, possible alternative approaches to drug therapy and so forth. Such activities may frequently include reviewing or following the patient in the patient care setting by means of the medical record chart and through consultation with the physician.

Education. This aspect of the service includes in-service and continuing education through formal lectures and informal discussions given to nurses, physicians, pharmacists, other health professionals and patients/consumers. This role is often extended to other areas, such as the hospital pharmacy and therapeutics committees, where the review of new and old drugs is undertaken by stressing documented proof of therapeutic merit, reports of adverse or untoward reactions and by making an appraisal of the merits of the drug in question relative to similar drugs. Another educational activity is the regular publication of a newsletter or bulletin which emphasizes the promotion of rational therapeutics by providing current information on new and old drugs and modes of therapy. In some cases, when a drug information service is affiliated with a college or school, the service may also be involved in the training of undergraduate and graduate students in the area of drug information.

It should be noted that drug information services are primarily patient-oriented and do not usually provide library-oriented services, such as retrieving or photocopying journal articles or compiling bibliographies for people engaged in research on problems unrelated to patient care.

Scope

Formal drug information centers generally attempt to provide health professionals with accurate, unbiased information on drugs, and specialize in recommending specific solutions to patient related drug problems. Services are usually provided on a 24 hours a day, seven days a week basis. Less formal services or satellite centers need not be based on such a schedule. When a drug information service is affiliated with satellite centers, it then serves as a backup resource for its affiliates. The relationship of a community pharmacy which provides drug information to a larger regional or medical center drug information service is an appropriate example of this.

Activities

Administrative activities necessary for the smooth operation of the service include:
1. Developing operational policies;
2. Developing operational site communication systems, etc.;
3. Acquiring and maintaining accurate, up-to-date information resources, which include texts, journals, indexing systems;
4. Advertising the service and the access to it;
5. Maintaining records and reports generated by the service; and
6. Training, up-grading and supervising staff and other personnel.

The main emphasis of the drug information service is the effective and efficient processing of drug information requests in response to patient-oriented problems. This includes:
1. Receiving the request in a complete and clear form via the telephone, in person, or in writing (e.g., mail requests). This necessitates obtaining and organizing essential information (including patient histories and other background information) from the questioner, in order that the inquiry is clearly defined;

2. Interpreting the question and defining the specific areas which are to be researched;

3. Systematically, thoroughly and efficiently completing the necessary research related to the request;

4. Evaluating the literature in an accurate, unbiased manner;

5. Formulating a relevant, coherent and informative response; and

6. Communicating the response clearly in an oral and/or written form using an appropriate format and documentation.

Drug information services may function as an educational *entity* in a number of ways which include:

1. The formal education and training of undergraduate, postgraduate and health professional students in the specialty area of drug information;

2. Providing continuing education programs, seminars and lectures on drug topics to the health professional communities on various drug related topics/subjects;

3. Providing consumer information to the public directly through patient counseling, through presentations or lectures to civic or other groups or through articles appearing in lay publications; and

4. Writing, editing, or publishing articles promoting a philosophy of rational drug therapeutics:

a. Publishing in appropriate professional journals, either as original or review articles or as regular feature columns; or

b. Publishing a regular newsletter/bulletin which the service organizes, edits and publishes as a means to promote an open communication on drug therapy. Such a newsletter may include:

(1) Drug reviews and evaluations;

(2) Drug literature abstracts and reports;

(3) Adverse reactions reports; and

(4) Interesting consultations provided by the service.

Drug information services are usually provided by clinically trained pharmacists. These pharmacists have received a clinically-oriented education with courses in pathology, drug therapeutics and pharmacokinetics, as well as clinical clerkships. Although not always necessary, an increasing number of pharmacists are graduating with Doctor of Pharmacy degrees (Pharm.D.) and are pursuing advanced postgraduate clinical training programs, i.e., residencies in clinical pharmacy. Incidentally, all residency programs accredited by the American Society of Hospital Pharmacists must offer training in drug information services. This clinical background enables the pharmacist to be selective and discriminating in providing drug information and to use critical judgement to assess the information available. Above all, the pharmacist is able to analyze and interpret the information, place it in the proper clinical perspective and communicate it in an effective manner to the user.

The clinically trained drug information specialist should be able to:

1. Locate sources of good clinical information from:
   a. General references and text books;
   b. Specialized information services such as abstracting services and indexing services; and
   c. Scientific and professional journals;
2. Interpret, analyze and evaluate this information objectively and accurately; and
3. Be able to communicate such information effectively, both verbally over the telephone, in person and/or in the form of written reports.

Depending upon the scope of coverage of a given drug information service, manpower requirements will vary. A small informal service usually requires a minimum of one pharmacist, but a major service may require more. It is generally accepted that in order to provide a seven day a week, twenty four hour a day service, about 4.2 full-time equivalent pharmacists are required. This figure does not account for administrative time, research and development time, vacation and sick leave time and high volume work loads. If time for these additional activities is included, the manpower estimates in Table 1 would serve as general guidelines for the staffing of a unit.

Table 1. Guidelines to Staffing a Drug Information Service

FUNCTION	FULL TIME EQUIVALENT PHARMACISTS
Twenty-four hour, seven day/week service	4.2
Administration	0.5–1.0
Publication of news bulletin	0.5–1.0
Pharmacy and Therapeutics committee & formulary	0.5–1.0
Research & development functions	0.5–1.0
Vacation & sick leave	0.6–1.0
Total	6.8–10.0

The approximations in this table are guidelines only and the requirements for a functioning drug information service may be greater or smaller, depending on the actual scope and workload of that service.

It may also be essential to have an adequate secretarial staff.

The secretarial staffing requirements will also vary with the service, but at least a part-time secretary will be necessary to carry out the administrative duties and the work generated by the service (e.g., typed requests, correspondence, bulletins).

Students, both at the undergraduate and graduate training levels, can be involved in providing drug information services. Although it is important to recognize that student involvement in the drug information service is primarily for educational experiences, with appropriate guidance and supervision students should be able to respond to information requests and consultations, prepare drug monographs and evaluations, prepare newsletters, bulletins or other publications and participate in certain administrative functions. These activities are part of the typical educational goals of the student. Other goals expect the student to:

1. Develop an appreciation of the skills, equipment, operating procedures and principles necessary to establish and maintain a drug information service;

2. Understand the position and role of drug information in the provision of total health care; and

3. Develop the student's individual skills in the collection, analysis and dissemination of drug information.

Location and Layout

The location and layout of a drug information service is often critical to its successful operation. The considerations are space availability, accessibility and scope of service. The parameters identified must be recognized as interdependent and the ultimate decision as to the final location of the drug information service revolves around all three aspects.

Space availability is a major consideration. In most cases, particularly in institutional settings, space is at a premium and is not easily obtained. In institutions such as hospitals or medical centers, formal requests for space may have to be initiated and presented in a justifiable manner to the appropriate administrators. In cases where the drug information service is to be a physical part of a pharmacy, space may sometimes be obtained by rearranging the physical structures. Efficient utilization of the space on hand may often provide an answer.

The accessibility of the service from the viewpoint of the user and the provider should be considered. From the viewpoint of the user of the service, its location should be convenient. Experience has shown that the utilization of a service is enhanced if it is in a location convenient to the user, e.g., close to patient care areas. From the viewpoint of the provider of drug information, the service should be located in an area where pharmacists can obtain information quickly, for example, within or adjacent to a medical library. If funds are not available to provide a full-time pharmacist to constantly man the drug information service, then its location should be convenient for all concerned, such as within the pharmacy, next to work areas or in close proximity to the pharmacy.

The scope of the service primarily dictates the space requirements. Needless to say, the larger the service provided, e.g., the greater the number of requests and consultations answered per day, the greater the space requirement. Very active operations, such as those serving a busy medical center or a large professional population, may require in excess of 400 square feet of operational space. Alternatively, drug information services serving a small number of health professionals and/or operating out of a community pharmacy may require only enough space to store the information resources adequately.

The location and layout of a service depend upon a number of variables and should be designed to meet the requirements and needs of each individual service's own situation. The literature provides examples of operational layouts for a large drug information service oriented to meeting the needs of a large institution (e.g., medical center or large hospital) and a small drug information service located within a pharmacy (e.g., a small community hospital or community pharmacy).

Background Reading

1. Blissit, C.W.: Consultations: The Drug Information Specialist *In* Blissit, C.W. et al. (Eds.), *Clinical Pharmacy Practice*, Lea and Febiger, Philadelphia, Pennsylvania, 1972, pp. 341–346

2. Burkholder, D.F.: Some Experiences in the Establishment and Operation of a Drug Information Center, *Am. J. Hosp. Pharm. 20*:506–513, 1963

3. Hirschman, J.L.: Building a Clinically-oriented Drug Information Service *In* Francke, D.E. and Whitney, H.A.K., Jr. (Eds.), *Perspectives in Clinical Pharmacy*, Drug Intelligence Publications, Hamilton, Il., 1972, pp. 159–160

4. Reilly, M.J.: *Drug Information: Literature Review of Needs, Resources and Services*. U.S. D.H.E.W., DHEW Public No. (HSM) 72-3013, Rockville, Maryland

5. King, C.M., Jr. et al.: *Drug Information Services: Two Operational Models*, U.S. D.H.E.W., DHEW Publ. No. (HSM) 72-3030, Rockville, Maryland

Integration of Poison Control and Drug Information Services

Many users of a drug information service consider drug information to be synonymous with poison control activities. While it may sometimes be said that a good drug information service also makes a good poison information service, or vice-versa, there are distinct differences. However, for all practical purposes, the overlap between the types of services provided by drug information and poison control is such that differences between the two become relatively minor. The following discussion points out the rationale for combining the two types of service.

The general manpower and staffing requirements for both services are essentially identical. Both may require a twenty-four hour a day, seven-day a week service capability. The type of individual staffing these services can usually be trained to handle both types of problem, providing they have had sufficient clinical background or training.

The information specialist functioning in either drug information and/or poison control must:

1. Be proficient in the retrieval, utilization and evaluation of the drug and poisoning literature;

2. Have had clinical experience in providing patient care in order to provide relevant and pertinent answers or information; and

3. Be able to communicate effectively, both in a verbal and written manner.

Both poison control and drug information services must maintain similar reference sources and materials. The purchase and maintenance of these resource materials represents a considerable investment—both as an initial expenditure and also as an annual expenditure to insure that all information is current. An integrated drug information and poison control service can utilize a majority of the same resource materials. This represents a substantial financial saving and makes a combined drug-poison information service a feasible consideration.

Since drug information services provide general information on drugs and recommend specific solutions to patient-related drug problems, a significant portion of drug information requests overlap with the types of information service provided by poison control centers. These include, but are not necessarily limited to, inquiries related to drug toxicities, adverse reactions and poisoning treatment, as well as to other aspects of the safe, therapeutic use of drugs. Other functions that both drug information and poison control services perform include the education and training of students, health professionals and the public by means of formal programs, presentations and publications.

The basic operational system for both drug and poison information services is similar. In either service, incoming requests or consultations are received at a central switchboard, either by telephone or by personal communication. After the problem has been completely identified, an answer pertinent to the request or problem is generated by staff personnel and communicated to the requestor. Thus, since the mechanism and resources for handling requests or problems already exists, the only requirement for a combined operational service would be the capability to respond to either type of information inquiry. This has been overcome in some instances by the use of clinical pharmacists who have had an education as well as a clinical training in both drug information and toxicology. The use of this type of personnel is advantageous not only from the standpoint of the quality of service, but also because the current direction of the pharmacy profession and pharmaceutical education make such trained individuals readily available.

In summary, the provision of drug information services with poison information or poison control services is both reasonable, appropriate and fiscally sound. The clinically trained pharmacist with appropriate experience and background has a definite role in the provision of drug and poison information.

The Systematic Approach:
A Discussion of the Concept

The changes occurring in professional pharmacy practice have been reflected in pharmacy education and curriculums, by an emphasis on drugs as agents which can elicit both therapeutic and adverse effects in patients. This patient-oriented pharmacy practice is also known as clinical pharmacy.

Most clinically-oriented pharmacists practice with the benefit of clinical experience; however, pharmacy students just beginning their clinical clerkships and experiences are often at a loss when approaching their new role because of their lack of "clinical experience." As a means of overcoming this deficiency, authors have advocated a systematic approach, with the instruction of students in basic practice concepts which can and will have future application

(Kishi and Watanabe, 1974; Watanabe et al., 1975). The systematic approach is the basis of this workbook-syllabus and is highly recommended as a technique for the fledgling clinical pharmacy student studying drug information skills. Since most practitioners rely on intuition, previous experience and often luck when answering drug information requests, the systematic approach will enable the student to initiate the formulation of a reasonable response without overlooking significant facts or resources. The following outline represents the principal points emphasized in this syllabus and is taken from Watanabe et al. (1975).

Background Reading

1. Kishi, D.T., and Watanabe, A.S.: A Systematic Approach to Drug Therapy for the Pharmacist, *Am. J. Hosp. Pharm.* 31:491–497, 1974
2. Watanabe, A.S. et al.: A Systematic Approach to Drug Information Requests, *Am J. Hosp. Pharm.*, 32:1282–1285, 1975

Training Protocol for Handling
Drug Information Requests

Step I
1. **Obtain caller's name, address, phone number and profession.**
2. **Classify the request and find out its nature,** i.e., what the caller thinks (s)he wants to know.

Step II **Obtain the necessary background information from the caller.**
1. **Is this request about a specific patient? If yes,** obtain:
   a. Patient's name, location, age, weight, sex;
   b. Patient's medical history summary;
   c. Patient's major organ functions (cardiac, kidney, liver, G.I., endocrine, etc.);
   d. Patient's drug history—prescription and OTC (name, dose, regimen, duration, indication); and
   e. Patient's history of allergy or adverse drug reaction; **if positive** obtain drug, description of reaction, route of exposure, date, treatment.
2. **Obtain other pertinent data specific to the request** (cf. appropriate request classification protocol in Chapter 3).
3. **Has questioner or caller searched any reference sources?** If yes, obtain citings.

Step III **Systematic Search**
1. **Begin the search by examining the available reference texts.** If the request concerns a topic (e.g., drug, disease state, etc.) that is unfamiliar, select a basic background text and research the topic *generally* before beginning a more specific search.

2. If an adequate answer cannot be found in the general references, **proceed to the secondary reference sources** listed for the appropriate request classification protocol. Often, these sources will provide an answer, or at the very least give a primary reference citing which can be consulted.

3. If an answer cannot be found using secondary reference sources, **the primary reference must be searched for** (i.e., the original reference or journal article). Primary reference source citings may be obtained from (1) general textbooks; (2) secondary reference sources or specific journals that are known to be useful for the given subject area of the question.

p IV Formulate a response pertinent to the request and the circumstances of the request. Be sure that all statements and conclusions are accurate and that the appropriate documentation is noted, i.e., each and every answer or statement should be traceable in the literature. Generally speaking, unreferenced statements (regardless of how obvious they may seem) are of very little value to the service. For written consultation responses, the following outline should be helpful.

1. **Request and background information.** This should be a brief statement of the problem and its circumstances.

2. **Response.**
   a. *Introduction.* In some cases a brief introductory opening is necessary for clarification of the terminology, issues at hand, etc.
   b. *Findings.* Summarize what the literature says about the problem. Any inadequacies or deficiencies of the studies and references cited should also be noted. Be concise, unbiased and, above all, accurate.
   c. *Tables, graphs, charts.* Include where appropriate any tables, graphs and charts (original or otherwise) that will assist and clarify the literature findings.

3. **Conclusion.** Briefly summarize the information found, together with the appropriate conclusions. This portion of the response should answer the request—everything written in the findings should merely substantiate the answer or conclusion. In addition, this portion of the response should include any recommendations, alterations, adjustments, etc. in the management of the questioner's problems.

4. **References.** All significant and important statements in the main body of the report should be referenced. To re-emphasize: any unreferenced statement of fact is for all practical purposes useless. Reference citings should follow the standard format.
   a. *Books.*
      Chapter Author(s): Chapter Title *In* Author(s)/Editor(s), *Book Title,* Edition, Publisher, year, pages
   b. *Journals.*
      Author(s): Title of article, *Journal name and volume:* pages (month) year

ep V Follow-up
Whenever possible, follow-up procedures should be undertaken either by phone call, in person or by mail. This is done in order to determine:

1. If the right question was in fact asked and the right answer was given;
2. If the answer was accepted and if an impact was made on patient care; and
3. If further assistance can be given.

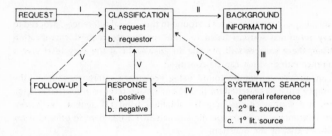

Figure 1. Systematic Approach to Answering Drug Information Requests

From Watanabe, A.S. et al.: Am. J. Hosp. Pharm. 32:1284, 1975. Reproduced with permission

Self Evaluation Questions For Introduction to Drug Information Concepts

1.1 Each individual must determine his or her own professional goals and objectives. Define your own professional aspirations and goals, i.e., how you would like your future pharmacy practice to be.

1.2 Indicate innovative ideas on how you can apply drug information skills to your future practice (as described in question 1.1). Attempt to envision specific examples and point out how you can offer similar services to those offered by drug information centers.

1.3 Attempt to envision or describe how you would promote yourself as a drug information specialist, in order to convince others of the value and utility of your skills.

1.4 Describe the systematic approach to drug information requests.

1.5 Identify the importance of a systematic approach in providing poison and drug information.

2

How to Classify a Request

Behavioral Objectives

General Discussion

Rationale

Types of classifications

Self Evaluation Questions and Learning Examples

Behavioral Objectives for Chapter Two
How to Classify a Request

OBJECTIVE	CRITERIA FOR MEETING OBJECTIVE	SELF EVALUATION QUESTION NUMBER
The student should be able to:		
2.1 Demonstrate skills for receiving and classifying a request in a logical order	2.1 Develop an understanding for the implications of classifying requests with respect to the following points: 2.2.1 Obtaining background information and history 2.2.2 Searching the literature 2.2.3 Providing an answer	2.2

	2.2 Obtain from the caller the necessary information to receive and classify requests; necessary information to include:
	2.1.1 Source of call
	    2.1.11 Consumer
	    2.1.12 Health professional
	    2.1.13 If health professional, type of affiliation, e.g., M.D., Pharm.D., D.D.S., D.V.M., R.N., R.Ph.
	    2.1.14 Speciality or type of practice, e.g., hospital vs. community, general practice vs. pediatrics
		2.1

continued

Behavioral Objectives for Chapter Two
How to Classify a Request (*continued*)

OBJECTIVE	CRITERIA FOR MEETING OBJECTIVE	SELF EVALUATION QUESTION NUMBER
2.1 Demonstrate skills for receiving and classifying a request in a logical order (continued)	2.3 Obtain necessary information to classify a request.	
	2.2.1 Pharmaceutical	2.3
	2.2.11 Availability	
	2.2.12 Identification	
	2.2.13 Compatibility	
	2.2.2 Drug Dosing	2.4
	2.2.3 Drug Interaction	2.8
	2.2.4 Adverse Reaction	2.5
	2.2.5 Poisoning	2.7
	2.2.6 Drug Therapy or Efficacy	2.6
	2.2.7 Pharmacokinetics	

General Discussion

As emphasized in Chapter One, the key to providing accurate, useful drug and poison information is to initiate a systematic process or approach. The first step is to classify the request, either mentally or, more formally, on paper (see King et al. and Figures 1 and 2).

Rationale

The primary reason for classifying a request is to provide a foundation for the logical steps that follow in the systematic approach. This concept is particularly important for students who are without the benefit of experience in providing drug information. The specific reasons for classifying a request are to initiate thought processes and organize the researcher. They can be enumerated as follows:

1. Classifying a request aids in determining what further type of background or patient history information is required to identify the nature of the request correctly;

2. Classifying a request directs one to anticipate the preliminary reference sources that it will be necessary to search; and

3. Classification of the request will also determine the type and sophistication of response or answer to be generated.

Types of Classifications

Classification of the request can be broken down into two areas:

1. Nature of the request; and
2. Professional background of the requestor or caller.

The nature of the request is usually further broken down into simple or basic categories. A number of classification schemes have been advocated in the literature. However, the method of classification usually varies with the inclination of the individual and/or the service. There are no hard and fast rules for classifying requests. A

ROCKY MOUNTAIN DRUG CONSULTATION CENTER
REQUEST FORM

TIME_____   DATE_____   REPORT NO._____

REQUESTOR'S NAME_____   PROFESSION_____

ADDRESS_____

CITY/STATE/ZIP_____   TELEPHONE_____

NATURE OF REQUEST:
   Pharmaceutical _____   Pharmacokinetics_____   Dosing _____
   Adverse Reaction_____   Drug Therapy _____   Drug Interaction_____
                           Other _____

DESCRIPTION OF REQUEST

_____

_____

_____

Patient/Background Data: Age_____   Weight_____   Sex_____

   Drug History/Allergies_____

_____

Cardiac_____
Gastro. Intest._____
Liver_____
Endocrine_____
Kidney_____
Other_____

REQUESTOR INFORMATION

   Has caller searched answer/if so where?

   Response needed by: TIME_____DATE_____

   Written Answer   Yes_____ No_____   SEARCH INCLUDED:
   Received by_____   A. General References_____
   Response Given By_____   B. Iowa_____
   Time_____ Date_____   C. de Haen_____
                             D. InPharma_____
                             E. Other_____

Figure 1. An Example of a Drug Consultation Center Request Form

Inquirer: _____

Address: _____

_____

Phone: _____

Date: _____

**ROCKY MOUNTAIN DRUG
CONSULTATION CENTER**
Denver Department of Health & Hospitals
W. 8th and Cherokee
Denver, Colorado 80204
Telephone: 629-1204

DRUG CONSULTATION REPORT

Signature	Title	Date

A Cooperative Service of Univ. of Colorado School of Pharmacy/Denver Dept. of Health & Hospitals

Figure 2 An Example of a Drug Consultation Center Report Form

good example of a relatively simple scheme is given in Table 1 and in Figure 1 (a DCC Request Form). Most services utilize these categories for the purpose of maintaining statistical records of the service's workload. From an individual's viewpoint, classifying the request tips the individual off to the points listed previously. For example, a request for the identification of an unknown or unfamiliar drug should, upon classification by the pharmacist, first indicate what should be solicited from the caller with respect to the appropriate background information or further history surrounding the circumstances of the call. Secondly, the classification of the request should give an indication of the specific reference sources that will need to be consulted. The references that need to be consulted in order to identify an unknown or unfamiliar drug are not necessarily the same, and are most likely completely different, from the references required for other types of request classifications. Thirdly, classification of the request will give clues as to the type of answer required. That is, certain types of requests or questions will require only brief, simple responses, while others may require lengthy, complex answers.

The professional background of the requestor or caller can give similar insights. Calls or requests taken from physicians may require lengthy research in numerous areas, followed by a long involved response. Facts given to physicians may also require adequate documentation and referencing. Conversely, requests from other health care personnel do not usually require such in depth procedures and simple answers taken from one or two sources are often adequate. Another consideration is the area of practice or the speciality of the professional. Background information solicited from, or responses given to, pharmacists in the community often differs greatly from that solicited from, or given to, pharmacists practicing in hospital settings. Similarly, responses given to general practice physicians may require a different perspective than those given to specialists such as neurologists, pediatricians, etc.

In conclusion, classifying the request at the time it is received gives the pharmacist an immediate insight and clear understanding

Table I. Classification Categories for Drug Information Requests

Adverse Drug Reaction
Drug Dosing
Drug Interaction
Drug of Choice/Therapeutic Efficacy
Pharmaceutical Identification/Availability
Pharmacokinetics
Poisonings

of the nature of the call and how it should be approached. Tipoffs for the approach include those for: (1) soliciting the appropriate history and background information for the type of question; (2) identifying the preliminary areas of research or references and (3) identifying the type and sophistication of answer that will be required. The student should keep in mind that these are primarily concepts that will initiate an organized, systematic approach to answering the request.

Background Reading

1. Hirschman, J.L.: Building a Clinically-Oriented Drug Information Service In Francke, D.E. and Whitney, H.A.K., Jr. (Eds.), *Perspectives in Clinical Pharmacy,* Drug Intelligence Publication, Hamilton, Ill., 1972, p. 159

2. Watanabe, A.S. et al.: A Systematic Approach to Drug Information Requests, *Am. J. Hosp. Pharm.* 32:1282–1285, 1975

3. King, C.M., Jr. et al.: *Drug Information Services: Two Operational Models,* U.S.D.H.W., DHEW Publ. No. (HSM)72-3030, Rockville, Maryland

Self Evaluation Questions and Learning Examples on How to Classify a Request

2.1 Identify three classification criteria that should be considered after receiving an information call.

2.2 Identify the reasons and/or importance of classifying a request as it relates to the systematic search.

Learning Examples

Classify the following requests and identify other considerations in so classifying them.

2.3 A physician working in an obstetrics and gynecology clinic calls you to find out what is in FEP cream.

2.4 A nurse in the local hospital calls and asks you if a patient receiving a dose of 7.5 g of chloramphenicol (Chloromycetin®) every six hours is reasonable.

2.5 A D.D.S. calls in asking about one of his patients who experiences drowsiness after receiving an injection of a local anesthetic.

2.6 Another pharmacist in a nearby pharmacy calls you about a prescription he has received about the use of neutral red for a herpes viral condition and wants to know if it is appropriate to dispense it.

2.7 A distraught mother calls and tells you that her daughter has taken a number of tablets used to treat their fish aquarium.

2.8 A local physician calls you and says that one of his patients has been taking Norflex® and some Darvon® and is now experiencing some unusual side effects. Classify this request and identify the necessity for classifying this request.

3

How to Obtain History and Background Information

Behavioral Objectives

General Discussion

The Patient's Medical History

The Patient's Drug or Medication History

Background Information

Self Evaluation Questions and Learning Examples

Behavioral Objectives For Chapter Three
How to Obtain History and Background Information

OBJECTIVE	CRITERIA FOR MEETING OBJECTIVE	SELF EVALUATION QUESTION NUMBER
The student should be able to:		
3.1 Demonstrate skills in taking a medical history	3.1 Obtain an accurate and complete medical history with regard to the circumstances of a request. This will require:	
	3.1.1 Information on the specific patient, to include:	3.1
	3.1.11 Patient's name, age, weight, sex	
	3.1.12 Patient's medical history summary	
	3.1.13 Patient's major organ functions (cardiac, kidney, liver, etc.)	
	3.1.14 Patient's drug history	
	3.1.15 Patient's drug allergy/adverse reaction history	
	3.1.2 Information specific to the request classification	3.2 3.5
3.2 Demonstrate skills in taking a complete drug history	3.2 Obtain an accurate and complete history regarding the patient's past and present prescription and non-prescription medications. This will require:	3.2 3.5
	3.2.1 For prescription and non-prescription medications:	
	3.2.11 Name of drug	

continued

Behavioral Objectives For Chapter Three
How to Obtain History and Background Information
(*continued*)

OBJECTIVE	CRITERIA FOR MEETING OBJECTIVE	SELF EVALUATION QUESTION NUMBER
3.2 Demonstrate skills in taking a complete drug history (continued)	3.2.12 Dosage and dosing regimen 3.2.13 Route of administration 3.2.14 Duration of therapy 3.2.15 Indication 3.2.2 Past medications the patient is not currently taking 3.2.3 Adverse drug reaction/drug allergy history 3.2.31 Drug, dosage, route of administration, indication 3.2.32 Date, description and treatment of reaction 3.2.33 Assessment of reaction	
3.3 Demonstrate skills in obtaining background information for specific request classifications	3.3 Obtain the following specific information for each request classification: 3.3.1 Pharmaceutical identification 3.2.11 Drug's country of origin 3.2.12 Drug's trade, generic, and/or chemical name 3.2.13 Drug's therapeutic use 3.2.14 Drug's manufacturer 3.2.15 Available dosage forms and description	3.3 3.5

continued

Behavioral Objectives For Chapter Three
How to Obtain History and Background Information
(continued)

OBJECTIVE	CRITERIA FOR MEETING OBJECTIVE	SELF EVALUATION QUESTION NUMBER
3.3 Demonstrate skills in obtaining background information for specific request classifications (continued)	3.2.16 Reason for inquiry	
	3.2.17 Reference source for this drug's inquiry	
	3.3.2 Drug Dosing	3.3
	3.3.21 Diagnosis/indication for which drug is prescribed	3.5
	3.3.22 Patient history (cf. 3.1)	
	3.3.23 Patient drug history (3.2)	
	3.3.3 Drug Interactions	3.3
	3.3.31 Specific interacting drugs	3.5
	3.3.32 Details of the suspected interaction	
	3.3.33 Patient history (cf, 3.1)	
	3.3.34 Patient drug history (cf. 3.3)	
	3.3.35 Management of the interaction	
	3.3.4 Adverse Reaction	3.3
	3.3.31 Description of adverse reaction	3.5
	3.3.32 Management of the reaction	
	3.3.33 Patient history (cf. 3.1)	
	3.3.34 Patient drug history (cf. 3.2)	

continued

Behavioral Objectives For Chapter Three
How to Obtain History and Background Information
(*continued*)

OBJECTIVE	CRITERIA FOR MEETING OBJECTIVE	SELF EVALUATION QUESTION NUMBER
3.3 Demonstrate skills in obtaining background information for specific request classifications (continued)	3.3.5 Poisoning	3.3
	3.3.51 Mode of exposure: ingestion, inhalation, percutaneous, ocular, envenomation, other	3.5
	3.3.52 Type of exposure: accidental, suicidal, environmental, drug abuse, other	
	3.3.53 Substance involved in exposure: Name and manufacturer, ingredients, amount involved, time since exposure	
	3.3.54 Status of victim: identifying features (age, weight, sex), present condition of victim (normal/asymptomatic or abnormal/symptomatic), present symptoms	
	3.3.55 Additional management data, including prior treatment(s), lab work results, supportive measures instituted	

continued

Behavioral Objectives For Chapter Three
How to Obtain History and Background Information
(continued)

OBJECTIVE	CRITERIA FOR MEETING OBJECTIVE	SELF EVALUATION QUESTION NUMBER
3.3 Demonstrate skills in obtaining background information for specific request classifications (continued)	3.3.6 Drug Therapy/Efficacy 3.3.61 Patient history (cf. 3.1) 3.3.62 Patient drug history (cf. 3.2)	3.3 3.5
3.4 Demonstrate an ability to determine the true nature of request by using the above skills		3.4 3.5
3.5 Be able to utilize information obtained from the history to place the answer in proper clinical perspective		3.4 3.5

General Discussion

The second step of the systematic approach is to obtain the necessary background and/or patient history information from the caller. Patient history information usually concerns itself with the pertinent medical considerations of a particular patient, i.e., the state and condition of the patient involved in the request. It should be noted that not all drug or poison information calls or requests involve a specific patient; however, when a specific patient is involved, then an adequate patient history must be obtained. In addition, a good history taken by the pharmacist will always include the patient's drug history.

Background information seeks further specifics concerning the circumstances and/or nature of the request and will include the patient's medical and drug history.

The importance of taking a history is well understood by physicians and nurses, but why should a pharmacist have such skills? The reasons may be many, but from the point of providing drug information there are two:

1. To give the pharmacist a better understanding of the actual request and the circumstances of the request, in order that (s)he may search for and provide a response; and

2. To enable the pharmacist to provide a more useful response and one that is appropriate to the specific clinical circumstances of the request.

The first reason requires an ability on the part of the pharmacist to determine what the caller wants to know, rather than what (s)he thinks (s)he wants to know. Often a caller may ask the pharmacist a question such as "what is the dosage of drug Y?" Without further information a completely accurate answer is impossible. The caller has not provided information such as:

1. Who is to receive this drug (i.e., age, sex, weight of the patient);

2. The status of the patient (health, vital organ functions);

3. The drug/medication history; and

4. The indication or therapeutic use of the drug.

Unless the pharmacist solicits additional information about this request, an inappropriate response may be given. The caller has asked only a part or a fragment of the actual question that requires a response. It may turn out upon further questioning, that the real question should have been, "Does the dosage of drug Y require adjustment in renal disease?" Alternatively, the caller may have asked the wrong question. An example of this would be when the caller asks, "What is the dosage of drug Y?", when what is really required is "What is the toxic dose of Y?", with reference to a patient who has acutely ingested a large amount of drug Y. Similarly, a caller may ask, "Is there any interaction between drugs A and B?", when what may actually be occurring is an interaction between other drugs or, alternatively, between a drug and a disease state. In these situations, the practical saying "Never assume anything" holds true; the pharmacist must always determine for him/herself the true nature of the caller's request by soliciting the appropriate history and background information.

The second important reason for the pharmacist to be able to obtain the history and background information is so that this information can be applied when formulating an answer or response. This requires the pharmacist to utilize his/her knowledge, clinical insight and judgement. To provide an answer to the previous example, the pharmacist must have information about the circumstances of the call, since the factors of age (infant, child, adult or geriatric), weight (lean, obese, etc.), health status (healthy, debilitated), vital organ function (kidney, liver function), drug history (drug interactions) and indication (proper, improper), are all major considerations in providing an appropriate response. Of course, an answer may be given without the additional background information and history, but the key to providing a more useful answer lies in the pharmacist's ability to obtain a good history and the necessary background information and to combine this with the insight to use the information and place the answer into its proper clinical perspective. It requires little or no ability to parrot a response from a standard reference source, but it is a reflection of true professional ability and practice to provide "tailor made" (i.e., pharmacist made) information to each individual request.

The ability to obtain appropriate history and background information requires considerable practice and only through practice will the student become proficient. It should be noted that history taking is considered by some to be more of an art than a science, and that each individual practitioner must determine what works best for him/herself. However, in order to provide an initial guideline for the student and to point out the basic requirements for obtaining history and background information, the following outline examples may be helpful.

The Patient's Medical History

Most information requests concern a specific patient, but the caller may or may not identify this fact. Therefore, the pharmacist must ask, "Does this request concern a specific patient?" If the response is yes, then the following additional questions must be asked of the caller.

What is the patient's age, sex and weight?

The pharmacist must be aware that age, sex and weight are definite considerations in providing information on drugs. Specifics may vary depending on the type (i.e., classification) of the request, but generally it is important to know if the request concerns a male or female, infant, adult, or geriatric and if the patient is lean, obese, etc.

Summarize the patient's medical history

A brief review of the patient's medical problems, diagnosis, etc., is required in order to gain a better understanding of the complete clinical situation of the patient. Certain disease states can and do alter drug action in the body and therefore require consideration.

What are the patient's major organ functions (including cardiac, kidney, liver, gastrointestinal, endocrine, etc)?

These may overlap with point two, but the reiteration is important. It is known that certain vital organ status or functions can and do affect a drug's action in the body. Very important considerations are renal and liver function, since these two routes are critical in drug elimination.

The Patient's Drug or Medication History

From a pharmacist's point of view, this is equally as important as the patient's medical history. The drug history can provide an insight into possible drug interactions and other such information. After obtaining the medical history, a drug history should be obtained as follows.

What prescription medications is the patient receiving?

This information should include the name of the drug (proprietary/tradename/generic), the dosage, the dosing regimen, route of administration, duration of therapy and indication. It is also useful to determine if the patient has received medications in the past which are not currently being taken.

What nonprescription (OTC) medications is the patient receiving?

This information is often overlooked but is an important consideration for the pharmacist. Although OTC drug use is usually significant only in chronic use or abuse and in overdose or poisoning situations, information for each specific medication should be obtained as for prescription medications.

Has the patient ever had an allergic reaction or adverse reaction to any medication?

The value of this question should be obvious; however, the concept of drug allergy or hypersensitivity is too often confused by patients and others with adverse reactions or side effects of drugs. Therefore, the pharmacist should obtain enough information about the reaction to be able to assess the reaction or side effect. This information should include:

1. *Drug name.* The most common categories of offenders are penicillins, sulfa and local anesthetics. The specific agent (trade name and/or generic name) should be solicited whenever possible.

2. *Drug dosage.* This is not always obtainable, but if available it may be helpful in differentiating between true hypersensitivity and adverse side effects resulting from inappropriate or usual dosages.

3. *Route of administration.* This is important since drug allergy occurs much more frequently by the parenteral route than by the oral route.

4. *Drug indication.* The reason why the drug was administered may give insight to the reaction.

5. *Description of the reaction.* An accurate, symptomatic description can often give an indication of the nature of the reaction (allergy vs. adverse) and its severity. Significant hypersensitivity symptoms are rash, urticaria, periorbital edema, shortness of breath, shock and loss of consciousness.

6. *Date of reaction.* An estimation of when the reaction occurred may be useful. Reactions that have occurred ten or twenty years ago may or may not be as clinically significant as a reaction occurring a few months ago.

7. *Treatment of the reaction.* Determining what was done to treat

the reaction may also give insight into the reaction's nature and severity.

Background Information

As noted previously, an important part of the background information of a patient related request is the patient's medical and drug history. However, other circumstances surrounding a request are important and require the pharmacist's consideration. Certain background information is specific to the type of request.

The following guidelines are based on the request classifications used in Chapter Two. With experience and thought, the student should be able to modify these guidelines to suit each individual request.

Pharmaceutical Identification

When a request concerns the identity of an unfamiliar drug, it is helpful for the pharmacist to obtain as many clues as possible to assist in identifying the unknown agent. The following questions are structured to obtain this type of background information.

What is the drug's country of origin?

This question will often be unnecessary but it is useful in determining where to look for an answer when a request deals with a foreign drug.

What is the drug's trade name and/or generic and/or chemical name?

If possible, when encountering a totally unfamiliar drug, an attempt to obtain all three names should be made. If its identity cannot be made using the trade or generic name, the chemical name will often yield results. Obviously correct spelling is critical, although not always possible. Consideration should be given in every case to other drugs with similar and/or different spelling before confirming an identity. Differentiation between prescription (legend) drugs and nonprescription (OTC) drugs should also be made.

What is this drug used for therapeutically?

An idea of a drug's use can also assist in establishing its identity. Two drugs spelt similarly can often be differentiated if their specific therapeutic use is known.

Which is this drug's manufacturer?

The identity of the manufacturer can also provide clues to a drug's identity. When all research possibilities are exhausted, the manufacturer can sometimes provide assistance.

In what dosage form is this drug available?

Physical characteristics and markings, as well as the specific types of dosage forms available (oral vs. parenteral; tablet vs. capsule, suppository, etc.), may provide clues to its identity.

What is the reference source of this drug?

Often identification inquiries come from patients via their physicians. It is important to know if the drug name came from word of mouth of the patient or from a label. Sometimes new, investigational, or foreign drugs are asked about as a result of their being mentioned in journal articles. In these cases, the specific journal or reference citation should be obtained for referral.

What is the reason for this inquiry?

This question will assist the pharmacist in determining what additional information should be provided. For example, if the inquiry concerns a foreign drug, an American equivalent may be necessary. If the real reason behind the inquiry is that a patient has ingested a large amount of the drug, poisoning information will be required.

Drug Dosing

Drug dosing questions usually lend themselves to rather simple answers straight from textbooks. Needless to say, such information may or may not be appropriate for a given patient. Thus, a number of considerations to the patient should be made and the following questions are structured to bring out these points.

What is the diagnosis or indication for which the drug is being prescribed?

Although the indication(s) for a drug may appear to be obvious, it is generally unwise to assume this fact. New indications for drugs are being discovered regularly and often require different dosing regimens. In addition, old dosing regimens are being re-evaluated and changed, e.g., as a result of the advent of drug serum level monitoring.

What is the age, sex and weight of the patient (include surface area, nutritional state, i.e., lean or obese, when appropriate)?

Most dosing requirements are based on weight (usually mg per kilogram of body weight). Age should definitely be a consideration, since pediatric and geriatric dosages are different to those for normal adults.

What is the status of the patient's renal and liver function (this usually requires recent, specific laboratory values)?

This information can be solicited in an adequate patient history, but it is mentioned again to re-emphasize the importance of being aware that renal and liver function status are vital determinants of appropriate dosage requirements.

What other medications is the patient taking now and has taken recently (i.e., in the last six months)? Does the patient have any known drug allergies?

This information should be solicited in the drug history but it is mentioned again here for purposes of thoroughness. It is known that certain drugs may interact and thus affect dosing requirements. In addition, it is obviously not wise to administer a drug to a patient who has in the past exhibited an allergic and/or severe adverse reaction to the drug being considered.

Drug Interactions

Drug interaction queries also lend themselves to simple answers. Such answers are assisted by the overabundance of charts, tables and reference texts on the subject. The pharmacist should be aware, however, that each situation requires individual consideration and that drug interactions may or may not occur, depending on the clinical circumstances. The following background questions are also useful when applied, with suitable modification, to drug-lab test interaction or modification queries.

What are the specific drugs in question?

The caller usually volunteers the drugs (s)he thinks are the interacting combination. As a result, the pharmacist should be cautious in assuming that the drugs mentioned by the caller are the only ones potentially causing the interactions. If the question concerns a laboratory test modification, then the laboratory test method should be obtained. Certain drug-lab test interactions are laboratory method specific.

What are the respective doses, duration of therapy and time course of administration of the drugs in question?

This question will assess the circumstances of the alleged interactions, pertinent laboratory values and the time sequence of consequences if they have not been administered together for a sufficient period of time, or in adequate dosages.

What are the details of the events secondary to the suspected action?

This includes the clinical symptoms or manifestations of the interactions, pertinent laboratory values and the time sequence of the occurring events as related to drug administration. An accurate description of the results of the interaction is required, in order to assess the nature of the interaction.

What is the current medical status of the patient?

The patient history is sometimes useful in assessing drug interactions, since certain drug-disease interactions may contribute to, or be mistaken for, drug-drug interactions.

What has been done to date in the management of this interaction?

This information may help determine what appropriate recommendations for the management of the drug interaction should be made.

Drug Therapy

Drug therapy questions cover a broad spectrum, ranging from drug of choice inquiries to comparative therapeutic efficacy evaluations. The advent of the pharmacist's involvement in the drug prescribing processes means that a good ability to handle this type of request is required. Such questions may or may not involve specific patients. When they do, the following background information is necessary, for reasons which have been discussed previously.

What is the age, sex, weight and race or nationality of the patient?

What is (are) the indication(s) and/or diagnosis in this patient? What other disease states does the patient have?

Include past medical history and surgical history.

What are the patient's current renal and liver functions?

Obtain the appropriate laboratory values.

What medications (both prescription and nonprescription/OTC) is the patient taking currently and has (s)he taken in the recent past?

Obtain the dose, duration, route of administration and indications for each drug.

Has the patient experienced any allergic and/or adverse reactions to medications in the past?

If so, obtain an appropriate history.

Adverse Drug Reactions

Questions relating to the adverse effect(s) of a drug or of combinations of drugs are a frequent occurrence and a cause and effect relationship between a drug and a reaction cannot always be established. However, the pharmacist can give some perspective when answering these types of requests. The following questions can assist in this endeavor. The first three questions are aimed at eliciting a complete description of the suspected adverse reaction.

What are the signs and symptoms of the possible adverse reaction?

Subjective and objective clinical findings should be included. Accurate descriptions are mandatory, since a statement such as "rash" is meaningless, due to the wide variety of rashes found. Laboratory values, both normal and abnormal, are useful descriptive parameters.

How severe is the reaction?

Information from this question may be highly subjective, but may provide insight to the nature of the reaction, e.g., "anaphylaxis associated with bronchospasm and edema" compared to "rash".

When did the reaction first become apparent?

Attempt to determine a temporal relationship between drug administration and the onset of the adverse reaction. Often this type of information is most useful in determining a cause and effect relationship. Without the specific time sequence of events, an accurate assessment is difficult.

What medications (both prescription and nonprescription) is the patient taking now and has (s)he taken during the past six months?

Obtain dose, duration, route of administration, and indication for each drug.

By now the importance of a good drug history should be well understood. Without this information, the possibility of drug-drug interactions, drug-lab test interactions and other potential offending agents cannot be excluded.

Has the patient or any member of the patient's family experienced any allergic and/or adverse reactions to medications in the past, especially one of a similar nature?

The past occurrence of an adverse or allergic reaction to a drug of an identical or similar nature in the patient, or even in a member of the patient's family, may provide indirect proof of a cause and effect relationship.

What is the current medical status of the patient?

Include diagnosis, renal function, liver function, age, sex, weight, race or nationality, etc.

It is known that certain patient-dependent conditions such as vital organ function, pharmacogenetics, etc., can and do effect the occurrence and severity of adverse drug reactions. Any and all such factors require consideration by the pharmacist.

What has been done in the management of the patient so far?

This information will influence what recommendations need to be made for the management of any adverse reaction. Some reactions are potentially life threatening and require immediate discontinuation of the offending agent, together with appropriate supportive therapy.

Poisoning

Obtaining a good history for calls concerning poisoning and ingestion may mean the difference between life and death. It is imperative that a definitive identification of the agent involved is obtained, together with enough history to assess its potential toxicity. The following questions should obtain most of the pertinent information.

What is the patient's age, weight and sex?

Age and weight are the critical determinants needed to assess the potential severity of the ingestion or exposure.

What is the alleged drug or chemical involved?

An accurate description of the compound is mandatory, and should include the trade name, generic or chemical names, together with a listing of ingredients for combination products, and the manufacturer's name. Correct identification of the ingested material is of primary importance, in order to assess the toxicity of the agent. The dosage form should also be considered, since oral solutions would be expected to be absorbed more quickly than solid forms.

What amount of the agent was ingested?

This is one of the most important pieces of information to obtain. In many cases, only rough estimates of the amount ingested will be available. Clues, such as the amount originally in the container, the amount remaining, the amount accountable by spillage, etc., may provide some insight, however. This information becomes critical when exposure to an agent at low doses is relatively safe, but exposure at higher doses is toxic.

How long ago was the agent ingested?

An estimation of the time elapsed since ingestion is necessary, as this will give some idea of what symptoms may be expected and it will also determine any necessary management procedures.

Were any other drugs, chemicals, or compounds also ingested?

This type of question may seem self evident, but it is best to search out all possible information. In a large number of drug ingestion cases alcohol is also involved, and multiple agent ingestions are not infrequent.

What was the route of exposure or administration?

Other routes beside the oral one are not uncommon and may include exposure via intravenous, cutaneous and ocular routes, or by inhalation. The severity of an ingestion or poisoning is often dictated by its route of exposure.

Does the patient have any acute or chronic diseases?

This question is often easily overlooked, since in most cases it has very little bearing on the prognosis or outcome of the ingestion.

However, certain pathological states, e.g., hepatic and renal function, may have a significant influence and should therefore be ascertained.

What symptoms is the patient exhibiting?

This question alone may not solicit all the symptomatology the patient is demonstrating. Often more specific questions pertinent to the type of ingestion and dealing with each organ system may be necessary (e.g., review of systems method, starting with the head (CNS) and working downward).

What has been done to treat the patient up to this time?

This question is another that often goes unasked. It is important to find out what has been done to determine both the immediate and future treatment modalities. Unfortunately, well wishers may initiate inappropriate measures which may complicate the situation. Hence, the importance of this last question.

Background Reading

1. Closson, R.: Foreign Drug Identification, *Drug Intell. Clin. Pharm.* 8:437–443, 1974

2. Davis, N.M.: Drug Information Requests: The Top of the Iceberg, *Hosp. Pharm.* 5:4, 1970

3. Hirschman, J.L. and Maudlin, R.K.: The DIAS Rounds, *Drug Intell. Clin. Pharm.* 4:45–48, 1970

4. Oderda, G.M. and West, S.: Emetics and Antiemetic Products, *In* Griffenhagen, G.B. and Hawkins, L.L. (Eds.), *Handbook of Nonprescription Drugs,* 5th Ed., American Pharmaceutical Association, Washington, D.C., 1977, p. 56

5. Shimomura, S.K. and Watanabe, A.S.: Adverse Drug Reactions, *Drug Intell. Clin. Pharm.* 9:190–197, 1975

Self Evaluation Questions and Learning Examples on How to Obtain History and Background Information

3.1 Indicate six considerations the pharmacist should make when obtaining the history and background information for a drug information request about a specific patient.

3.2 Indicate the considerations and information necessary for a complete drug history.

3.3 Identify specific pertinent background information for the following types of questions.

Pharmaceutical identification   Adverse reaction
Drug dosing   Poisoning
Drug interactions   Drug therapy/efficacy

3.4 Indicate two reasons why it is important for the pharmacist to be able to obtain history and background information.

3.5 *Learning Examples:* Identify the additional background and history information required to answer the following case examples adequately.

a. A physician requests the U.S. equivalent to an analgesic he used while in Europe. The drug is diamorphine.

b. A nurse calls and asks what the maximum daily intravenous dose of tetracycline is.

c. You receive a call from a physician who asks if there is an interaction between rifampin and coumarin anticoagulants and if it is important.

d. Another pharmacist calls to ask you if glycerol has been used in cerebral edema and, if so, how it should be given.

e. A physician calls and gives you the following information: A pediatric patient recently developed salmonella gastroenteritis and was treated with chloramphenicol. Within 48 hours from the initiation of chloramphenicol therapy she developed shock, respiratory difficulties, green diarrhea, an ashen color and became acidotic. He asks you if this can be a manifestation of the gray baby syndrome, which usually only occurs in children less than one month old.

f. *Patient History.* We have a 60-year-old 65 kg female who underwent gastroscopy and was premedicated with Demerol® 25 mg IV x 2, followed with 2.5 mg Valium® IV. The patient was also on Donnatal® as an outpatient but has not received or taken any for 24 hours. She has no known allergies. Liver and kidney function are normal. Shortly after receiving the premedications at 9:00 a.m., the patient became rigid and arched her back but without any tonic or clonic movements. Her pupils were widely dilated and she became apneic with a drop in heart rate to 38 beats per minute. She was treated with oxygen, and transferred to the ICU. At 11:30 she had a second apneic episode with a heart rate of 30–50.

Request: Is this an allergic reaction to Demerol®? Can she be treated with naloxone, i.e., if this is an allergic reaction, will there be any risk of further exacerbation due to cross allergenicity of naloxone and Demerol®?

4

How to Conduct a Systematic
Literature Search

Behavioral Objectives

General Discussion

Literature Hierarchy

Classification Tables of References

Self Evaluation Questions and Learning Examples

Behavioral Objectives for Chapter Four
How to Conduct a Systematic Literature Search

OBJECTIVE	CRITERIA FOR MEETING OBJECTIVE	SELF EVALUATION QUESTION NUMBER
The student should be able to:		
4.1 Demonstrate skills for retrieval of necessary information	4.1.1 Discuss the rationale behind a systematic literature search method	4.1
4.2 Demonstrate awareness and familiarity with available information resources and their appropriate use	4.2.1 Define and describe the terms general, secondary and primary reference sources	4.2
	4.2.2 Identify by title and author or editor, general, secondary and primary reference sources	
	4.2.3 Identify the use of each reference source and the type of information available from each source	
4.3 Demonstrate an ability to conduct a thorough, systematic search of the literature	4.3.1 Identify a logical sequence for initiating and completing a search	4.3 4.4
	4.2.11 General reference sources	
	4.2.12 Secondary reference sources	
	4.2.12 Primary reference sources	

General Discussion

The third step of the systematic approach is to initiate a search of the literature. Most clinical practitioners are able to conduct a literature search in a competent manner as a result of their professional training and clinical experiences. However, students or pharmacists without the benefit of previous experience in researching the literature often have difficulty in initiating a search, or determining how to conduct a thorough search. In most cases, a good search requires (1) a basic familiarity with the available information sources and (2) an organized methodology in covering these available sources. This is the systematic search (see Figure 1).

Although most practitioners have individualized their literature retrieval and search techniques to suit their own personal needs, the systematic search is designed to (1) show the inexperienced student how to conduct a thorough and complete review of the informational sources and (2) provide a foundation on which the student is able to develop personalized search techniques. In essence, the systematic search technique is designed to prevent the student from overlooking significant facts and/or reference sources.

Literature Hierarchy

An awareness of the basic information sources is required to conduct a systematic search. The student should be familiar with

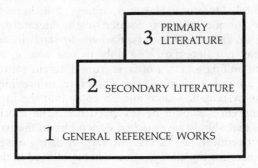

Figure 1. The Steps of the Systematic Search of the Literature Hierarchy

the three types or classes of information sources in the literature hierarchy, as outlined by Walton et al. (Blisset, *Clin. Pharm. Practice*). They are as follows.

General Reference Works

The student is probably already familiar with this classification of information sources. These sources present documented information in a condensed and compact format which arises from a background of publications from the primary literature. Examples include textbooks, general reference books, review articles and compilations.

Secondary Literature

These sources are intermediate between the general reference sources and the primary literature. They represent a group of heterogeneous information sources that function as a guide or direct line to the primary literature. They are available in a number of different formats, such as abstracting services, bibliographic listings and specialized microfilm or microfiche systems. Examples of the most commonly used systems are listed in Table I.

Primary Literature

Primary literature includes journal publications dealing with scientific and nonscientific data with a particular emphasis on drug related subjects, such as reports of clinical drug trials, case reports, pharmacologic research, etc. The primary literature is the foundation on which the previous literature classifications are based.

With an adequate understanding of the types of information sources available, the student should be prepared to initiate a search of the literature. However, unless it is known precisely where the specific answer is located in the literature, it may be confusing or difficult to ascertain where to start. In addition, an answer may not necessarily be only in one source, and it may require the pulling together of facts from different sources and the review of a number of references. Therefore, to provide the initial step of the systematic search and an entry into the literature, the general references should be reviewed first. The specific general references that should be searched depend upon the nature of the question or request, i.e., its classification. A listing of specific general references for the classification scheme utilized in this syllabus appears in the tables at the end of this discussion. It should be noted that these tables are not necessarily meant to be all inclusive, but are merely provided as initial guidelines.

If an adequate answer cannot be generated from the general references alone, or a more indepth or thorough response is required, the next step in the systematic search is to review the secondary reference sources. The indexing, abstracting and other specialized services and systems may provide enough information for an adequate response, or at the very least may provide reference citations to the primary literature. Secondary reference sources are not necessarily restricted in their scope to certain types of information. Exceptions, however, are *Adverse Reaction Titles* from the Excerpta Medica Foundation, *Clin Alert* from Science Editors, Inc. and *Toxicity Bibliography* from *Index Medicus* of the National Library of Medicine. These sources are more specific for information on the adverse reactions and toxicity of drugs.

The primary literature is the third step of the systematic search and the most specific source of information. A review of the primary literature with an emphasis on the most current and up-to-date citations and facts is required in all responses of an extensive or indepth nature. Examples of this would include drug therapy reviews or evaluations, adverse drug reactions, or current dosing regimens or techniques. Depending on the specific subject or nature of the request, subspeciality journals in the primary literature may be referred to directly. For example, pediatric journals may be referred to for pediatric related requests, cancer journals for questions related to cancer therapy, etc. (see Allyn, 1976).

In addition, it is helpful for the pharmacist searching the primary literature to know how far back in time it is necessary to look for reference citations. For example, a pharmacist receives a question regarding a drug-drug interaction. It may be of limited value to research the literature beyond the early 1960's, since most drug interactions were not fully recognized until after the mid-to-late 1960's. Similarly, if a question on the mechanism of action of triamterene was received, it would be most helpful to know that triamterene (Dyazide®) was introduced by Smith, Kline and French in 1964. Therefore, the pharmacist must search the primary literature just prior to 1964, as well as after that time, in order to do a complete and thorough job. For relatively new drugs, e.g., naproxen, which was introduced in 1976, searching the literature before the latter part of the 1960's may be an inefficient use of time. Paul de Haen recently compiled a convenient list of drugs and the year they were introduced, dating from 1940 through to 1975 (de Haen, 1976 and 1978).

Background Reading

1. Allyn, R.: The Literature of Medicine: A Library for Internists II, *Ann. Intern. Med. 84*:346–373, 1976

2. Brandon, A.N.: Selected List of Books and Journals for the Small Medical Library, *Bull. Med. Libr. Assoc. 59*:266–285, 1971

3. de Haen, P.: Compilation of New Drugs: 1940 through 1975, *Pharm. Times:* 40–74 (Mar.) 1976

4. Walton, C.A. et al.: Drug Literature Utilization: Selection, Evaluation, and Communication *In* Blissett, C.M. et al. (Eds.), *Clinical Pharmacy Practice*, Lea and Febiger, Philadelphia, Pa., 1972, pp. 374–406

5. Watanabe, A.S. et al.: A Systematic Approach to Drug Information Requests, *Am. J. Hosp. Pharm. 32*:1282–1285, 1975

6. de Haen, P.: *de Haen Nonproprietary Name Index*, Volume X -1977, Paul de Haen, Inc., New York, N.Y., 1978

Classification Tables of Reference

Table A. References Useful in Answering Drug Identification and Availability Requests

REFERENCE	INFORMATION

General References

REFERENCE	INFORMATION
American Druggist: *Blue Book 1978*, Hearst Corporation, New York, N.Y., 1978	Tablet and capsule ID; availability; manufacturer
American Hospital Formulary Service (AHFS), American Society of Hospital Pharmacists, Washington, D.C.	Availability; formulations
Anon.: *APhA Drug Names*, American Pharmaceutical Association, Washington, D.C., 1976	Proprietary and nonproprietary names and manufacturers
Anon.: *Unlisted Drugs Index-Guide/4* Unlisted Drugs, Chatham, N.J., 1977	Drugs in research; drug ID; drug code numbers; synonyms
Billups, N.F.: *American Drug Index*, J.B. Lippincott Co., Philadelphia, Pa., 1978	Availability; manufacturer; not all drugs in ADI are marketed, i.e., investigational
Canadian Drug Identification Code, 2nd Ed., Drug Information Division, Bureau of Drug Surveillance, Drugs Directorate, Health Protection Branch, Dept. of National Health and Welfare, Canada	Canadian drug ID
Collier, W.A.L.: *Imprex*, 7th Edition, Donald Ferrier Ltd., Edinburgh, Scotland. Distributed by Drug Intelligence Publications, Inc., Hamilton, Il., 1978	Index of imprints on tablets and capsules from U.S.A. and U.K. and many other countries worldwide
Compendium of Pharmaceutical Specialities (CPS), 13th Ed., Canadian Pharmaceutical Association, Toronto, Canada, 1978	Canadian and French drug ID
Drug Topics Red Book 1977, Medical Economics Company, Oradell, N.J., 1977	Availability; tablet and capsule ID; manufacturer

continued

Table A. References Useful in Answering Drug
Identification and Availability Requests (*continued*)

REFERENCE	INFORMATION
Penna, R.P. and Kleinfeld, C. (Eds.): *Handbook of Nonprescription Drugs*, American Pharmaceutical Association, Washington, D.C., 1977	OTC drug availability and ID
Griffiths, M.C. (Ed.): *USAN and the USP Dictionary of Drug Names*, United States Pharmacopeial Convention, Inc., Rockville, Md., issued annually	Identification; foreign drugs; manufacturer
Index Nominum, Swiss Society of Pharmacy, Zurich, Switzerland, 1978, issued every two years. Distributed by Drug Intelligence Publications, Inc., Hamilton, Il.	Investigational and foreign drug ID
Kastrup, E.K.: *Facts and Comparisons*, Facts and Comparisons, Inc., St. Louis, Mo. (updated monthly)	Availability; new drugs; formulations; useful lists of comparable agents
Marler, E.E.J.: *Pharmacological and Chemical Synonyms*, Excerpta Medica, Amsterdam, 1976	Investigational and foreign drug ID
National Drug Code Directory, Volumes 1 & 2, Office of Scientific Coordination, Bureau of Drugs, Food and Drug Administration, Department of Health, Education and Welfare, Washington, D.C., 1976	Tablet and capsule ID; availability; manufacturer
Negwer, M.: *Organisch-Chemische Arzneimittel und ihre Synonyma*, Akademie-Verlag, Berlin, 1978. Distributed by Verlag Chemie, New York City and Drug Intelligence Publications, Inc., Hamilton, Il.	Investigational and foreign drug ID
Pharm-Index, Skyline Publishers, Inc., Portland, Or. (monthly supplements)	Availability; new drugs; manufacturer. Investigational drug index section
Physicians Desk Reference (PDR), Medical Economics Co., Oradell, N.J., (annual)	Tablet/capsule ID
Rosenstein, E. (Ed.): *Diccionario de Especialidades Farmaceuticas*, 23rd Ed., P.L.M., S.A. Medellin No. 184 Mexico 7. Distributed by Drug Intelligence Publications, Inc., Hamilton, Il., 1977	Mexican and other foreign drugs

Table A. (*continued*)

REFERENCE	INFORMATION
Rumack, B.H. (Ed.): *Poisindex*, Micromedex, Inc., Rocky Mountain Poison Center, Denver, Co. (updated quarterly)	Ingredients of products, tablet & capsule ID
Stecher, P.G. (Ed.): *Merck Index*, 9th Ed., Merck & Co., Inc., Rahway, N.J., 1976	Chemical names; foreign drugs
Wade, A. (Ed.): *Martindale—The Extra Pharmacopoeia*, 27th Ed., The Pharmaceutical Press, London, 1977. Distributed by Rittenhouse Book Distributors, Inc., Philadelphia, Pa. and Drug Intelligence Publications, Inc., Hamilton, Il.	Availability; major drugs; investigational drugs; formulation; manufacturer

Secondary References

de Haen Drugs in Research, Paul de Haen, Inc., New York, N.Y.	Investigational and foreign drug ID
de Haen Drugs in Use, Paul de Haen, Inc., New York, N.Y.	Investigational and foreign drug ID
Unlisted Drugs, Pharmaco-Medical Documentation, Box 401, Chatham, N.J.	Investigational and foreign drug ID

Other Sources

Compendia of the country of origin of the drug	Foreign drug ID
Specific manufacturers (the address and telephone numbers of drug manufacturers are listed in the *Physicians' Desk Reference* (PDR), *Bluebook*, *Redbook* and *American Drug Index*)	
The Food and Drug Administration	

Table B. General References Useful in Answering Drug Dosing Requests[a]

GENERAL REFERENCE	INFORMATION
AMA Drug Evaluations, 3rd Ed., American Medical Association, Chicago, Il., 1977	General dosing, (Recommended by AMA)
American Hospital Formulary Service (AHFS), American Society of Hospital Pharmacists, Washington, D.C.	General dosing
Anderson, R.J. et al.: *Clinical Use of Drugs in Renal Failure*, Charles C Thomas, Springfield, Il., 1976	Dosing in renal impairment, dialysis
Conn, H.F. (Ed.): *Current Therapy, 1978*, W.B. Saunders Co., Philadelphia, Pa., 1978	General dosing
Facts and Comparisons, Facts and Comparisons, Inc., St. Louis, Mo.	General dosing
Kempe, C.H. et al.: *Current Pediatric Diagnosis and Treatment*, 5th Ed., Lange Medical Publications, Los Altos, Ca., 1978	Pediatric dosing
Knoben, J.E. et al.: *Handbook of Clinical Drug Data*, 4th Ed., Drug Intelligence Publications, Inc., Hamilton Il., 1978	General dosing; dosing in pregnancy, geriatrics, renal impairment
Kucers, A., and Bennett, N.: *The Use of Antibiotics*, 2nd Ed., J.B. Lippincott Co., Philadelphia, Pa., 1975	Antibiotic dosing
Modell, W. (Ed.): *Drugs of Choice 1976–1977*, C.V. Mosby Co., St. Louis, Mo., 1976	Dosage in specific conditions
Osol, A. and Pratt, R.: *U.S. Dispensatory*, 27th Ed., J.B. Lippincott Co., Philadelphia, Pa., 1973	General dosing
Physicians' Desk Reference (PDR), Medical Economics Co., Oradell, N.J. (annual)	General dosing only, manufacturers' recommendations
Reidenberg, M.M.: *Renal Function and Drug Action*, W.B. Saunders Co., Philadelphia, Pa., 1971	Dose in renal impairment
Shirkey, H.C.: *Pediatric Dosage Handbook*, American Pharmaceutical Association, Washington, D.C., 1973	Pediatric dosing

Table B. (*continued*)

GENERAL REFERENCE	INFORMATION
Shirkey, H.C. (Ed.): *Pediatric Therapy*, 5th Ed., C.V. Mosby Co., St. Louis, Mo., 1975	Pediatric dosing
Shirkey, H.C.: *Pediatric Drug Handbook*, W.B. Saunders Co., Philadelphia, Pa., 1977	Pediatric dosing
Standard Pharmacology Textbooks	General dosing
The Harriet Lane Handbook, Year Book Medical Publications, Chicago, Il.	Pediatric dosing
Wade, A. (Ed.): *Martindale—The Extra Pharmacopoeia*, 27th Ed., The Pharmaceutical Press, London, 1977. Distributed by Rittenhouse Book Distributors, Inc., Philadelphia, Pa. and Drug Intelligence Publications, Inc., Hamilton, Il.	General dosing

[a]Refer to Specialized Texts for dosing in specific disease states

Table C. General References Useful in Answering Drug
Interaction Requests/Laboratory Test Interferences
and IV Incompatibilities

REFERENCE	INFORMATION

General References

Cohen, S.N. and Armstrong, M.F., *Drug Interactions: A Handbook for Clinical Use*, Williams and Wilkins Co., Baltimore, Md., 1974	Drug-drug interaction monographs with references
Cohon, M.: *Intravenous Incompatibilities*, University of Wisconsin Hospitals, Madison, Wi., 1974	IV Incompatibilities
Cohon, M: *Therapeutic Drug Interactions*, University of Wisconsin Medical Center, Madison, Wi. 1970	Drug-drug interaction
Constantine, N.V. and Kabat, H.F: Drug Induced Modifications of Laboratory Test Values—Revised 1973, *Am.J.Hosp.Pharm.30:* 24–71, 1973	Drug-lab
D'Arcy, P.F. and Griffin, J.P.: *A Manual of Adverse Drug Interactions*, John Wright and Sons, Ltd., Bristol, U.K., 1975	Drug-drug; table format
Drug Interactions-2, American Society of Hospital Pharmacists, Inc., Washington, D.C., 1973	Abstracts from IPA on drug interactions
Evaluations of Drug Interactions, 2nd Ed., (APhA) and yearly supplement, American Pharmaceutical Association, Washington, D.C. 1976	Drug-drug interaction monographs; well referenced
Francke, D.E., and Whitney, H. A. K., Jr. (Eds.): *Perspectives in Clinical Pharmacy*, Drug Intelligence Publications, Hamilton, Il., 1972	IV Incompatibilities
Gahart, Betty L.: *Intravenous Medications—A Handbook for Nurses and Other Allied Health Personnel*, C.V. Mosby Co., St. Louis, Mo., 1975	IV Incompatibilities
Garb, S.: *Clinical Guide to Undesirable Drug Interactions and Interferences*, Springer Publishing Co., Inc., New York, N.Y., 1971	Drug-drug, drug-lab test (Tabulation and References)

Table C. (*continued*)

REFERENCE	INFORMATION
Hansten, P.D.: *Drug Interactions,* 3rd Ed., Lea and Febiger, Philadelphia, Pa., 1975	Most useful, well documented drug-drug and drug-lab interaction monographs
Hartshorn, E.A.: *Handbook of Drug Interactions,* 3rd Ed. Drug Intelligence Publications, Inc., Hamilton, Il., 1977	Drug-drug interaction, drug-lab test interferences
Interaction of Alcohol and Other Drugs, Addiction Research Foundation, Toronto, Ontario, Canada, 1972	Drugs with alcohol abstracts
King, J.C.: *Guide to Parenteral Admixtures,* Cutter Labs, Inc., St. Louis, Mo., 1970. Updated regularly	IV admixtures
Knoben, J.E. et al.: *Handbook of Clinical Drug Data,* 4th Ed., Drug Intelligence Publications, Inc., Hamilton, Il., 1978	Drug-drug; drug-lab (in tables)
Martin, E.W.: *Hazards of Medication,* 2nd Ed., J.B. Lippincott Co., Phila., Pa., 1978	Table-drug-drug interactions; drug-lab tests
Powers, S.: *Incompatibilities of Pre-op Medications,* Hospital Formulary Management, May, 1970	Interactions between pre-op medications
Sawyer, N. et al.: *Cross-Indexed Reference Manual of Human Drug Interactions,* University of Alabama, Birmingham, Al., 1971	Drug-drug interaction
Trissel, L.A.: *Handbook on Injectable Drugs,* American Society of Hospital Pharmacists, Washington, D.C., 1977	IV administration and admixture information by monographs; referenced
Trissel, L.A., Grimes, C.R. and Gallelli, J.F.: *Parenteral Drug Information Guide (ASHP),* American Society of Hospital Pharmacists, Washington, D.C., 1974	IV admixtures
Wade, A. (Ed.): *Martindale—The Extra Pharmacopoeia,* 27th Ed., The Pharmaceutical Press, London, 1977. Distributed by Rittenhouse Book Distributors, Inc., Philadelphia, Pa. and Drug Intelligence Publications, Inc., Hamilton, Il.	Abstracts on drug stability and compatibility
Young, D.S. et al.: *Effects of Drugs on Clinical Laboratory Tests,* Clinical Chemistry (Suppl.), Bethesda, Md., April, 1975	Drug-lab test

continued

Table C. General References Useful in Answering Drug Interaction Requests/Laboratory Test Interferences and IV Incompatibilities (*continued*)

REFERENCE	INFORMATION
Cluff, L.E. and Petrie, J.C.: *Clinical Effects of Interaction Between Drugs*, Excerpta Medica, Amsterdam, American Elsevier Publishing Co., Inc., New York, N.Y., 1974	General articles on drug interactions
Drug Interactions—An Annotated Bibliography, National Library of Medicine, United States Department of Health, Education & Welfare, Bethesda, Md.	Drug-drug, de Haen abstract format
Francke, D.E. (Ed.): *Handbooks of IV Additive Reviews, 1970, 1971, 1972, 1973*, Drug Intelligence Publications, Inc., Hamilton, Il.	Abstracts and articles on IV admixtures and incompatibilities

Secondary References

REFERENCE	INFORMATION
Adverse Reaction Titles, Excerpta Medica Foundation, Amsterdam	Abstracts, including rare and obscure drug interactions
Clin-Alert, Science Editors, Inc., Louisville, Ky.	Abstracts on drug-drug interactions from literature (400 journals)
de Haen Drugs in Use, Paul de Haen, Inc., New York, N.Y.	Abstracts drug-drug interactions
Index Medicus, National Library of Medicine, United States Department of Health, Education and Welfare, Bethesda, Md.	Abstracts
InPharma, Quarterly index and recent issues, ADIS press, New York, N.Y.	Current information as abstracts
Iowa Drug Information System, Iowa Drug Information Service, Iowa City, Iowa	Original articles

Table D. General References Useful in Answering Adverse Drug Reaction Requests

REFERENCE	INFORMATION
General References	
American Hospital Formulary Service (AHFS), American Society of Hospital Pharmacists, Washington D.C.	General
Cluff, L., Caranasos, G.J. and Stewart, R.B.: *Clinical Problems With Drugs*, Vol. 4, W.B. Saunders Co., Philadelphia, Pa., 1975	Tables and discussion for major reactions
D'Arcy, P.F. and Griffin, J.P.: *Iatrogenic Diseases*, Oxford University Press, London, 1972	General discussion by type of reaction
deGruchy, G.C.: *Drug-Induced Blood Disorders*, Blackwell Scientific Publications, London, 1975	Blood dyscrasia; chapters by type of dyscrasia
Dimitrov, N.V. and Nodine, J.H. (Eds.): *Drugs and Hematologic Reactions*, Grune and Stratton, New York, N.Y., 1974	Blood dyscrasia; effects listed by blood element
Dukes, M.N.G. (Ed.): *Side Effects of Drugs Annuals 1 and 2* Excerpta Medica, Amsterdam, Elsevier North Holland Inc., New York, N.Y., 1977 and 1978	Yearly supplement to *Side Effects of Drugs;* index to 2 is cumulative
Fraunfelder, F.T.: *Drug-Induced Ocular Side Effects and Drug Interactions*, Lea & Febiger, Philadelphia, Pa., 1976	Ocular effects listed by drug
Girdwood, R.H. (Ed.): *Blood Disorders due to Drugs and Other Agents*, Excerpta Medica, Amsterdam, 1974	General discussion, specific types of blood dyscrasia
Grant, W.M.: *Toxicology of the Eye*, 2nd Ed., Charles C Thomas, Springfield, Il., 1974	Adverse ocular effects of systemic drugs
Heinonem, O.P. et al.: *Birth Defects and Drugs in Pregnancy*, Publish. Sci. Group, Littleton, Ma., 1977	Discusses malformations by system and by drug class
Knoben, J.E. et al.: *Handbook of Clinical Drug Data*, 4th Ed., Drug Intelligence Publications, Inc., Hamilton, Il., 1978	Tables of drug-induced blood, skin, hepatic and renal reactions

continued

Table D. General References Useful in Answering Adverse
Drug Reaction Requests (*continued*)

REFERENCE	INFORMATION
Meyler, L. and Herxheimer, A.: *Side Effects of Drugs,* Vol. 4–8, The Williams and Wilkins Co., Baltimore, Maryland and Excerpta Medica Foundation, New York, N.Y.	General-cases; not cumulative, well referenced. First line reference
Meyler, L. and Peck, H.: *Drug-Induced Diseases,* Excerpta Medica, Amsterdam, 1972	Classification by organ system, well referenced
Miller, R.R. and Greenblatt, D.J. (Eds.): *Drug Effects in Hospitalized Patients,* John Wiley and Sons, New York, N.Y., 1976	Reports from Boston Collaborative Drug Surveillance team
Moser, R.H. (Ed.): *Diseases of Medical Progress: A Study of Iatrogenic Disease,* 3rd Ed., Charles C Thomas Publishers, Springfield, Il., 1969	General; well referenced
Shader, R.I. and DiMascio A. (Eds.): *Psychotropic Drug Side Effects: Clinical and Theoretical Perspectives,* Williams and Wilkins Co., Baltimore, Md., 1970	Reactions to all psychotropic agents by organ system
Shepard, T.H.: *Catalog of Teratogenic Agents,* The Johns Hopkins University Press, Baltimore, Md., 1973	Teratogenicity. Mostly animal reports. Good screening tool
Swanson, M. and Cook, R.: *Drugs, Chemicals, and Blood Dyscrasias,* Drug Intelligence Publications, Inc., Hamilton, Il., 1977	Listing of blood abnormalities due to drugs and chemicals
Tuchmann-Duplessis, H.: *Drug Effects on the Fetus,* Adis Press, Sydney, Australia, 1975	Teratogenicity; discussion and drug classes
Wade, A. (Ed.): *Martindale-The Extra Pharmacopoeia,* 27th Ed., The Pharmaceutical Press, London, 1977. Distributed by Rittenhouse Book Distributors, Inc., Philadelphia, Pa. and Drug Intelligence Publications, Inc., Hamilton, Il.	General, case abstracts

Secondary References

Adverse Reaction Titles, Excerpta Medica, Amsterdam	Monthly bibliography of adverse reactions from 3400 journals
Clin-Alert, Science Editors, Inc., Louisville, Ky. (biweekly)	Abstracts of adverse reactions from 400 journals

Table D. (*continued*)

REFERENCE	INFORMATION
de Haen Drugs in Use, Paul de Haen, Inc., New York, N.Y.	Abstracts on cards
FDA Clinical Experience Abstracts, Dept. of Health, Education and Welfare, Food and Drug Administration, Rockville, Md.	Abstracts on cards of adverse reactions
INPHARMA, Quarterly Index and recent issues, ADIS Press, New York, N.Y.	Abstracts from recent literature
Iowa Drug Information System, Iowa Drug Information Service, Iowa City, Ia.	Primary literature
Toxicity Bibliography, National Library of Medicine, United States Department of Health, Education and Welfare, Bethesda, Md.	Index to adverse reactions and poisonings (taken from data base of *Index Medicus*)

Table E. General References Useful in Answering Drug Therapy Efficacy Requests

General References

Accepted Dental Therapeutics, 36th Ed., American Dental Association, Chicago, Illinois, 1975

Avery, G.S. (Ed.): *Drug Treatment*, ADIS Press, New York, N.Y., 1976

Boedacker, E.C. (Ed.): *Manual of Medical Therapeutics*, 2nd Ed., Little, Brown and Co., Boston, Ma., 1977

Conn, H.F. (Ed.): *Current Therapy 1978*, W.B. Saunders Co., Philadelphia, Pennsylvania, 1978

Herfindal, E.T. and Hirschman, J.I. (Eds.): *Clinical Pharmacy and Therapeutics*, Williams and Wilkins Co., Baltimore, Md., 1975

Krupp, M.A. and Chatton, M.J. (Eds.): *Current Medical Diagnosis and Treatment*, Lange Medical Publications, Los Altos, Ca., 1978

Melmon, K.L. & Morelli, H.F. (Eds.): *Clinical Pharmacology*, 2nd Ed., The Macmillan Company, New York, N.Y., 1978

Modell, W. (Ed.): *Drugs of Choice 1978-1979*, C.V. Mosby Co., St. Louis, Mo., 1978

The Medical Letter on Drugs and Therapeutics, New Rochelle, N.Y.

Thorn, G.W., et al. (Eds.): *Harrison's Principles of Internal Medicine*, 8th Ed., McGraw-Hill Book Company, New York, N.Y., 1977

Wade, A. (Ed.): *Martindale—The Extra Pharmacopoeia*, 27th Ed., The Pharmaceutical Press, London, 1977. Distributed by Rittenhouse Book Distributors, Inc., Philadelphia, Pa. and Drug Intelligence Publications, Inc., Hamilton, Il.

Young, L.Y. and Kimble, M.A. (Eds.): *Applied Therapeutics for Clinical Pharmacists*, Applied Therapeutics, Inc., San Francisco, Ca., 1975

Standard pharmacology and medical textbooks

Secondary References

Current Contents-Clinical Practice, Institute for Scientific Information, Philadelphia, Pa. (subject index) current information

de Haen Drugs in Use, Paul de Haen, Inc., New York, New York, under specific drug in question

Index Medicus, National Library of Medicine, U.S. Department of Health, Education and Welfare, Washington, D.C., under the disease or drug name

Table E. (*continued*)

INPHARMA Quarterly Index, and recent issues, ADIS Press, New York, current information

Iowa Drug Information System, Iowa Drug Information Service, Iowa City, Iowa, under Disease State (ICDA) microfiche system

Medline Search

Other General References in Specialized Areas

Azarnoff, D.L. (Ed.): *Steroid Therapy,* W.B. Saunders Co., Philadelphia, Pa., 1975

Bondy, P.K. and Rosenberg, L.E. (Eds.): *Duncan's Diseases of Metabolism,* W.B. Saunders Co., Philadelphia, Pa., 1974

Garrod, L.P. et al.: *Antibiotic and Chemotherapy,* 4th Ed., Churchhill Livingstone, London, England, 1973

Greenblatt, D.J. and Shader, R.I.: *Benzodiazepines in Clinical Practice,* Raven Press, New York, N.Y., 1974

Havener, W.H.: *Ocular Pharmacology,* 3rd. Ed., C.V. Mosby Co., St. Louis, Missouri, 1974

Hollander, J.L. and McCarty, D.J. (Eds.): *Arthritis and Allied Conditions,* 8th Ed., Lea and Febiger, Philadelphia, Pa., 1972

Horton, J. and Hill, G.J.: *Clinical Oncology,* W.B. Saunders Co., Philadelphia, Pa., 1977

Kagan, B.M.: *Antimicrobial Therapy,* 2nd Ed., W.B. Saunders Co., Philadelphia, Pa., 1974

Klein, D.F. and Davis, J.M.: *Diagnosis and Treatment of Psychiatric Disorders,* Williams and Wilkins Co., Baltimore, Md., 1969

Kucers, A. and Bennett, N. Mck.: *The Use of Antibiotics,* 2nd Ed., William Heinemann Medical Books Ltd., London, England, 1975

Markell, E.K. and Voge, M.: *Medical Parasitology,* 3rd Ed., W.B. Saunders Co., Philadelphia, Pa., 1971

Medical Letter Handbook of Antimicrobial Therapy, The Medical Letter on Drugs and Therapeutics, New Rochelle, N.Y., 1974

Merritt, H.H.: *A Textbook of Neurology,* Lea and Febiger, Philadelphia, Pa., 1973

Mulholland, J.H. (Ed.): *Bugs and Drugs, 1976,* Bugs and Drugs, Inc., University City, Mo., 1976

Sauer, G.C.: *Manual of Skin Diseases,* J.B. Lippincott Co., Philadelphia, Pa., 1973

continued

Table E. General References Useful in Answering
Drug Therapy Efficacy Requests (*continued*)

Sherlock, S.: *Diseases of the Liver and Biliary System,* Blackwell Scientific Publications, Oxford, England, 1975

Woodbury, D.M., Penry, J.K. and Schmidt, R.P. (Eds.): *Antiepileptic Drugs,* Raven Press, New York, N.Y., 1972

Table F. General References Useful in Answering Pharmacokinetics Questions

REFERENCES	INFORMATION[a]
General References	
American Hospital Formulary Service (AHFS), American Society of Hospital Pharmacists, Washington, D.C.	ADME, $t_{1/2}$, serum levels
Anderson, P.O.: Drugs and Breast Feeding—A Review, *Drug Intell. Clin. Pharm.* 11:208, 1977	Drugs in breast milk; concentration and clinical effects
Anderson, R.J. et al.: *Clinical Use of Drugs in Renal Failure*, Charles C Thomas, Springfield, Il., 1975	Dosing in renal failure, ADME
Benet, L.Z. (Ed.): *The Effect of Disease States on Drug Pharmacokinetics*, American Pharmaceutical Association, Washington D.C., 1978	Effects of disease on ADME
Bennett, M.M. et al.: Guide to Drug Usage in Adult Patients with Impaired Renal Function. *Ann. Intern. Med. 86*:754–783, 1977	Dosing in renal failure; $t_{1/2}$
Goldstein, A., Aronow, L. and Kalman, S.M.: *Principles of Drug Action: The Basis of Pharmacology*, 2nd Ed., John Wiley and Sons, New York, N.Y., 1974	General principles
Goodman, L.S. and Gilman, A., (Eds.): *The Pharmacological Basis of Therapeutics*, 5th Ed., The Macmillan Co., New York, N.Y., 1975	ADME, $t_{1/2}$, serum levels
Jackson, F. and McLeod, D.: Pharmacokinetics and Dosing of Antimicrobials in Renal Impairment, *Am.J.Hosp.Pharm. 31*:36, 137, 1974	Dosing in renal failure
Knoben, J.E. et al.: *Handbook of Clinical Drug Data*, 4th Ed., Drug Intelligence Publications, Inc., Hamilton, Il., 1978	ADME, $t_{1/2}$, serum levels of commonly used drugs
Koch-Weser, J.: Serum Concentrations as Therapeutic Guides, *N.Engl.J.Med. 228*:227, 1972	Drug concentration levels
O'Brien, T.D.: Excretion of Drugs in Human Milk, *Am.J.Hosp.Pharm. 31*:844–854, 1974	Drugs in breast milk; concentration and clinical effects

continued

Table F. General References Useful in Answering Pharmacokinetics Questions (continued)

REFERENCES	INFORMATION[a]
Pagliaro, L.A. and Benet, L.Z.: Clinical Compilation of Terminal Half-lives, Percent Excreted Unchanged and Changes of Half-lives in Renal and Hepatic Dysfunction for Studies in Humans with References, *J.Pharmacokinet.Biopharm. 3:333–383, 1975*	As in article title
Paselt, R.C. et al.: Therapeutic and Toxic Concentrations of more than 100 Toxicologically Significant Drugs in Blood, Plasma, or Serum: A Tabulation, *Clin.Chem. 21:44–62, 1975*	Drug concentration levels
Reidenberg, M.M.: *Renal Function and Drug Action,* W.B. Saunders Co., Philadelphia, Pa., 1971	Dosing in renal failure; $t_{1/2}$
Ritschel, W.A.: pKa Values and some Clinical Applications, *In* Francke, D.E. and Whitney, H.A.K., Jr. (Eds.): *Perspectives in Clinical Pharmacy,* Drug Intelligence Publications, Inc., Hamilton, Il., 1972	pKa
Ritschel, W.A.: Biological Half-lives and Their Clinical Applications, *In* Francke, D.E. and Whitney, H.A.K., Jr. (Eds.): *Perspectives in Clinical Pharmacy,* Drug Intelligence Publications, Inc., Hamilton, Il., 1972	$t_{1/2}$
Ritschel, W.A.: *Handbook of Basic Pharmacokinetics,* 1st Ed., Drug Intelligence Publications, Inc., Hamilton, Il., 1976	General principles, ADME, $t_{1/2}$, data on important drugs
Rowland, M.: Drug Administration and Regimens, *In Clinical Pharmacology,* 2nd Ed. Melmon, K.L. and Morelli, H.F. (Eds.), The Macmillan Co., New York, N.Y., 1978	General principles
Simpson and Joergens: Biological Half-Life and Rational Drug Therapy, *Hosp. Pharm.,* 8:(Mar.) 1973	$t_{1/2}$
Standard Pharmacology Textbooks	General Information
Wade, A. (Ed.): *Martindale—The Extra Pharmacopoeia,* 27th Ed., The Pharmaceutical Press, London, 1977. Distributed by Rittenhouse Book Distributors, Inc., Philadelphia, Pa. and Drug Intelligence Publications, Inc., Hamilton, Il.	ADME, $t_{1/2}$

Table F. (*continued*)

REFERENCES	INFORMATION[a]
Wagner, J.G.: *Biopharmaceutics and Relevant Pharmacokinetics*, 1st Ed., Drug Intelligence Publications, Inc., Hamilton, Il., 1971	General principles
Wagner, J.G.: *Fundamentals of Clinical Pharmacokinetics*, Drug Intelligence Publications, Inc., Hamilton, Il., 1975	General principles
Woodbury, D.M., Penry, J.K., Schmidt, R.P. (Eds.): *Antiepileptic Drugs*, Raven Press, New York, N.Y., 1972	ADME, $t_{1/2}$, serum levels for anticonvulsant drugs

Secondary References

de Haen Drugs in Use, Paul de Haen Inc., New York, N.Y., Specific agent

Index Medicus, (new series) National Library of Medicine, United States Department of Health, Education and Welfare, Bethesda, Md.

INPHARMA, Quarterly Index and recent issues, ADIS Press, New York, N.Y.

Iowa Drug Information System, Iowa Drug Information Service, Iowa City, Ia., Specific Drug

[a] Abbreviations: ADME = absorption, distribution, metabolism, excretion
$t_{1/2}$ = Half-life

Table G. General References Useful in Answering
Poison Information Requests

GENERAL REFERENCE	INFORMATION
Anon.: *The Sinister Garden: A Guide to the Most Common Poisonous Plants*, Wyeth Labs, Philadelphia, Pa.	Symptoms and treatment for common poisonous plants; illustrated
Arena, J.: The Perils in Plants, *Emergency Medicine:* (Feb.) 1974	Listing of poisonous plants and treatment
Arena, J.: *Poisoning: Toxicology, Symptoms, Treatments*, 3rd Ed., Charles C Thomas, Springfield, Il., 1974	Categorical review of poisonous substances; good for identifying symptoms but not treatment
Browning, E.: *Toxic Solvents*, Edward Arnold & Co., London, England, 1972	Toxicity and treatment of industrial solvents
Christensen, H. et al.: *Toxic Substances List*, U.S. Dept. HEW, Public Health Service, Center for Disease Control, National Institute for Occupational Safety and Health, Rockville, Md.	List of toxic ingredients and other toxicological values (LD_{50}, MAC, etc.)
de Haen Drugs in Use, Paul de Haen, Inc., New York	Case studies (abstracts) of poisonings due to drugs
Deichman, W.B. and Gerarde, H.W.: *Toxicology of Drugs and Chemicals*, Acadium Press, New York, N.Y., 1969	Easy to use; alphabetical listing of toxic drugs and chemicals
Dreisbach, R.: *Handbook of Poisoning*, 9th Ed., Lange Medical Publications, Los Altos, Ca., 1977	Toxicity and treatment of poisonings; very complete but antidotes inaccurate in some cases
Ellis, M.D.: *Dangerous Plants, Snakes, Arthropods and Marine Life, Toxicity and Treatment*, Drug Intelligence Publications, Inc., Hamilton, Il., 1978	Toxicity and treatment for wide variety of poisonings; well illustrated in color
Fluit, T. and Cain, H.: *Emergency Treatment and Management*, 5th Ed., W.B. Saunders Company, Philadelphia, Pa.	Toxicity and treatment of specific poisons, as well as other emergency situations
Gosselin, R. et al.: *Clinical Toxicology of Commercial Products*, 4th Ed., Williams and Wilkins Co., Baltimore, Md., 1976	The most comprehensive text. Sections include trade name, generic/chemical name, and general formulations
Grant, W.: *Toxicology of the Eye.*, 2nd Ed., Charles C Thomas., Springfield, Il., 1974	Effects of drugs and chemicals on the eye

Table G. (*continued*)

GENERAL REFERENCE	INFORMATION
Hamilton, A. and Hardy, H.: *Industrial Toxicology*, 3rd Ed., Publishing Sciences Group, Acton, Mass., 1974	Toxicity of industrial products
Hardin, J. et al.: *Human Poisoning from Native and Cultivated Plants*, Duke University Press, Durham, N.C., 1973	Symptoms and treatment from poisonous plants
Harrington, H.D.: *Edible Native Plants of the Rocky Mountains*, University of New Mexico Press, Albuquerque, N.M.	Description of non-toxic plants; illustrated
Iowa Drug Information System; School of Pharmacy, Drug Information Service, University of Iowa, Iowa City, Ia.	Indexing system to articles of poisoning cases
Kaye, S.: *Handbook of Emergency Toxicology*, Charles C Thomas, Springfield, Il., 1970	Toxicity and treatment of drug and chemical poisoning; also assay and analysis techniques
Kingsbury, J.M.: *Poisonous Plants of the U.S. and Canada*, Prentice Hall, Englewood Clifts, N.J., 1964	Toxicity of plants; most complete plant textbook; lacks treatment; illustrated
Lampe, K.F. and Fagerstrom, R.: *Plant Toxicity and Dermatitis*, Williams and Wilkins Co., Baltimore, Md., 1968	Toxicity of plants; illustrated
Matthew, H. and Lawson, A.: *Treatment of Common Acute Poisonings*, 3rd Ed., Churchill-Livingstone, Edinburgh, U.K.	Symptoms and treatment of common poisonings
Polson, C.J. and Tattersale, R.: *Clinical Toxicology*, 2nd Ed., J.B. Lippincott, Philadelphia, Pa.	Poisoning cases; review of specific poisons. Best for more extensive data on chronic poisonings
Poison Control Center, National Clearinghouse for Poison Control Center, HEW, Public Health Service, Rockville, Md.	Cards listing symptoms and treatment for poisoning due to drugs and chemicals; updated yearly
Rumack, B.H. (Ed.): *POISINDEX* System; Micromedex Inc., Rocky Mountain Poison Center, Denver, Co.	Over 180,000 products, plants, chemicals, their toxicity and treatment; a microfiche system, updated quarterly
Sax, I.N.: *Dangerous Properties of Industrial Materials*, 4th Ed., Reinhold Publishing Corp., New York, N.Y.	Toxic properties and symptoms of industrial materials

continued

Table G. General References Useful in Answering Poison Information Requests (*continued*)

GENERAL REFERENCE	INFORMATION
Toxicity Bibliography, National Library of Medicine, DHEW, Bethesda, Md.	Bibliographical citations from *Index Medicus* on adverse reactions and toxicity
Wade, A. (Ed.): *Martindale—The Extra Pharmacopoeia*, The Pharmaceutical Press, London, 1977. Distributed by Rittenhouse Book Distributors, Inc., Philadelphia, Pa. and Drug Intelligence Publications, Inc., Hamilton, Il.	Abstracts of poisonings due to drugs and chemicals; symptoms and treatment

Table H. References Useful in Answering Requests on the Potassium, Sodium, Sugar, Alcohol and Vitamin Content of Medicinal Preparations

REFERENCE	INFORMATION
The White Sheet, Potassium Content of Selected Medicinals, Philips Roxane Labs., Inc. Columbus, Oh.	Potassium content of selected medicinals
Pearson, R.E. and Fish, K.H.: Potassium Content of Selected Medicines, Foods and Salt Substitutes, *Hosp. Pharm.* 6:6–9, 1971	Potassium content
Sodium in Medicinals: Tables of Sodium Values, 1973, San Francisco Heart Association, San Francisco, Ca.	Sodium content
Bosso, J.A. and Pearson, R.E.: Sugar content of Selected Liquid Medicinals, *Diabetes* 22:776, 1973	Sugar content
Anon.: Sugar-Free Liquid Preparations, *Am. Drug.* 175:24–26, 1977	Sugar free medicinals
Knoben, J.E. et al.: *Handbook of Clinical Drug Data,* 4th Ed., Drug Intelligence Publications, Inc., Hamilton, Il., 1978	Sodium content of selected medicinals; sugar-free pharmaceuticals; potassium content of foods
American Druggist: *Bluebook,* Hearst Corporation, New York, N. Y.	Sugar content
Kastrup, E.K. (Ed.): *Facts and Comparisons,* Facts and Comparisons, Inc., St. Louis, Mo.	Alcohol content
Petroni, N.C. and Cardoni, A.A.: Alcohol Content of Selected Liquid Medicinals, *Drug Ther.* 1:214–218, 1976	Alcohol content
Penna, R.P. and Kleinfeld, C. (Eds.): *Handbook of Nonprescription Drugs,* American Pharmaceutical Association, Washington D.C., 1977	Alcohol content
Documentia Geigy, Scientific Tables, Geigy Pharmaceuticals	Vitamin content of foods
Manufacturers' Product Literature	

Table I. Secondary Literature Sources[1]—Indexing and Abstracting Services

	YEARS COVERED	APPROXIMATE NUMBER OF JOURNALS	COST PER YEAR	APPROXIMATE LAG TIME	COMMENTS
Adverse Reaction Titles, Excerpta Medica Foundation	1966 to present	3500	$1720.00	6–12 months	An excellent indexing service to search for rare and obscure adverse drug reactions
Clin-Alert, Science Editors, Inc.	1962 to present	150	$42.00	1–6 weeks	*Clin-Alert* abstracts reports of adverse drug reactions, drug interactions, medico-legal pitfalls and related therapeutic hazards; it has a very short lag time compared to most other abstracting services
Current Contents Clinical Practice, (CCCP), Institute for Scientific Information, Inc.	1973 to present	700	$135.00	1–6 weeks	CCCP is a compilation of the table of contents of about 700 journals as they are released; it covers the 3–6 month lag time that most other indexing and abstracting services miss; it is also useful for keeping up with the current literature and sending for reprints
de Haen, Drugs in Use, Paul de Haen, Inc., New York (Other services provided by Paul de Haen include *Drugs in Research, Drugs in Prospect, Adverse Reaction Index, Drug Interaction Index, New Product Survey, Drugs in Combination*).	1964–present	450	$800.00	6–24 months	de Haen is the single best indexing and abstracting service for drug information use; it is convenient, covers a reasonable number of journals and spans a period of over 10 years

continued

Source	Coverage	Journals	Price	Time	Description
Drug Literature Index, Excerpta Medica Foundation	1969–present	3500	$2100.00	6–12 months	The large number of journals it indexes is both an advantage and a disadvantage; it ensures a thorough literature search, but it is time consuming in that a number of obscure or foreign reference sources must be sifted through
FDA Clinical Experience Abstracts, Food and Drug Administration	1963 to present	180	free	12–24 months	FDA CEA contains abstracts on adverse effects, hazards, and efficacy of drugs, devices and nutrients as well as on adverse effects of cosmetics, household chemicals, pesticides, and food additives
Index Medicus, (New series) National Library of Medicine	1960 to present	2300	$173.00	3–12 months	An indexing service which covers the entire spectrum of the medical literature and not just drugs; about 25 percent of the articles indexed are drug oriented. Available on microfiche or microfilm from Pergamon Press ($90–200.00)
INPHARMA, ADIS Press, 488 Madison Avenue, New York, N. Y.	1975–present	1700	$295.00	3 weeks to 6+ months	INPHARMA is the most recent secondary source available and probably the most useful (along with Current Contents) for searching the most recent literature; it presents abstracts weekly from international journals as well as bibliographies on major topics of interest; a quarterly index is supplied
International Pharmaceutical Abstracts, (IPA), American Society for Hospital Pharmacists	1964 to present	1000	$150.00	6–14 months	IPA is a semi-monthly journal which covers the pharmaceutical, clinical, economic and scientific aspects of drug literature

continued

Table I. Secondary Literature Sources[1]—Indexing and Abstracting Services (continued)

	YEARS COVERED	APPROXIMATE NUMBER OF JOURNALS	COST PER YEAR	APPROXIMATE LAG TIME	COMMENTS
Iowa Drug Information Service, Clinical and Drug Information Service of the College of Pharmacy, University of Iowa	1964–present	144	$900.00	3–12 months	The Iowa System can be used in conjunction with, or as a reasonable substitute for, the de Haen system; it has the added advantage of providing the complete article on microfiche rather than just an abstract
Pharmacology and Toxicology, Excerpta Medica Foundation	1962 to present	3500	$264.00	3–6 months	Utilizes nearly the same data base as Adverse Reaction Titles and Drug Literature Index
Science Citation Index, (SCI), Institute for Scientific Information, Inc.	1961 to present	2200	$1800.00	3–12 months	SCI is an international, interdisciplinary index to the literature of science, medicine, agriculture, technology and the behavioral sciences; it is primarily a citation index rather than a subject index, although a subject index (Permuterm Subject Index) is also available
Toxicity Bibliography, National Library of Medicine, DHEW, Bethesda, Md.	1968 to present	2300	$32.00	3–6 months	An indexing service covering adverse reactions and poisonings; it is taken from the same data base as Index Medicus. Available on-line as Toxline
Unlisted Drugs, Pharmaco Medical Documentation, Box 401, Chatham, N. J.	1949 to present		$140.00		A monthly publication which describes investigational and foreign drugs not listed in usual compendia

continued

POISINDEX, Micromedex Inc., Rocky Mountain Poison Center, Denver, Co.	1974– present	N/A	$1000.00	3–6 months	Computer-output microfiche system on toxic substances; consists of product index (over 180,000 products listed) and managements for treatment of each; also excellent for drug identification requests
DRUGDEX, Micromedex Inc., Rocky Mountain Drug Consultation Center, Denver, Co.	1978	N/A	Approx. $1800.00	3–6 months	Computer-output drug information system on microfiche; consists of Index Guide, drug evaluations and drug consults; drug information is in usable and easily retrievable form

[1] Adapted from Shimomura and Watanabe, 1975

Self Evaluation Questions and Learning Examples on How to Conduct a Systematic Literature Search

4.1 Identify two reasons for using a systematic literature search method.

4.2 Identify the literature hierarchy, citing three examples of each type of reference source, the use of each and the type of information available from these sources.

4.3 Identify the rationale and sequence for initiating and completing a thorough search of the literature.

4.3 *Learning Examples: Use of General References*
   Answer the following questions and list the reference where the answer was found. Only reference texts will be necessary as it is not necessary to use secondary sources or primary literature.

Identification

1. What is Cardioquin® generically? What are its claimed advantages over other salts of this drug?

2. What is Repo-Estratest®? Who makes it?

3. What is in F&D Mixture? How toxic is it?

Availability

1. Dr. Smith has read a recent article on the use of medrogestone, a progestational agent, and would like to obtain this drug. Is this drug available and what is the trade name and manufacturer?

2. Does Vontrol® come as a suppository?

3. Is cyproterone acetate obtainable in the U.S.? By whom?

Therapeutic Use

1. What is glyrol used for?

2. What is the drug of choice for chancroid? What dose?

3. Has glycerol been used in cerebral edema? State how it should be given.

4. What reference provides you with a tabular compilation of antibiotics of choice for selected organisms?

Dosage

1. What is the maximum daily IV dose of tetracycline? What are the main toxic effects that can be expected if this dose is exceeded?

2. What reference provides a tabular comparison of dosages of corticosteroids and what does this reference list as the approximate equivalency of dose in mg between dexamethasone and methylprednisolone?

3. How much phenobarbital would you recommend giving to a 3-year-old girl as a sedative?

4. Will kanamycin dosing be altered by peritoneal dialysis?

Adverse Effects

1. Dr. Great calls regarding his patient who has been suffering from episodes of apnea. The patient has been on Darvon®, Dilantin®, and Aerosporin®. What is happening?

2. Dr. Tremendous has a patient in his office with a maculopapular erythematous rash over most of his body and oozing bullous lesions around the mouth. His temperature is 101° F and he has been anorexic and dysphagic for three days. He has been taking dyphenylhydantoin 50 mg tid and phenobarbital 65 mg as a suppository bid for focal seizures. The physician is wondering if his condition is drug-induced. What do you think is the problem?

3. Has respiratory depression ever been reported from gentamicin therapy?

4. Can corticosteroids increase intracranial pressure?

Drug Interactions

1. Is there an interaction between rifampin and coumarin anticoagulants, and if so, how significant is it?

2. Can spironolactone interfere with urinary 17-hydroxycorticosteroid determinations?

3. What in your opinion is the best reference on drug interactions? Why? Are there any drawbacks to this publication?

Pharmaceutical Compatibility

1. A nurse calls with orders to add 1,000 units heparin to an IV of 1,000 ml D_5/W containing 80 mg gentamicin sulfate. Is this compatible?

2. Why does tetracycline in an IV precipitate Solu-Cortef®?

3. Can Valium® be mixed in an IV solution?

Metabolism and Excretion

1. Why can Vibramycin® be given once daily?

2. Is albumin metabolized after IV administration?

3. What reference provides tables of plasma half-lives of drugs?

4. How is ethambutol metabolized and excreted? Are dose reductions necessary in renal impairment?

4.4 *Learning Examples: Use of Secondary Sources*
Use only secondary literature sources to answer the following questions. The following systems should be used if they are available:
de Haen Drugs in Use;
Iowa Drug Information System Drug/Disease File;
FDA Abstracts;
Clin-Alert;
International Pharmaceutical Abstracts; and
InPharma.
Only a short answer is necessary. Cite the article references for your answers.

1. You receive a call from Dr. Smith who is hesitant to prescribe reserpine because of recent reports of carcinogenicity. Is there any evidence of this?

2. Dr. Jones has a patient who has been on phenylbutazone 400 mg/day for 15 days. She was admitted for treatment of thrombophlebitis. Admitting lab values were SGOT 72, SGPT 58, LDH 78, Alk. Phos. 20, Bili (conj.) 0.1, Bili (total) 0.4. She has been on no other medication. Is this a drug-induced hepatitis?

3. The patient is a 45-year-old male with malignant hypertension. He is diabetic and we are hesitant to continue the use of diazoxide. He has received 3 doses (300 mg each). Can diazoxide be used safely in diabetics? Do you recommend sodium nitroprus-

side? What dose should be given? The patient is also hypothyroid and stabilized on thyroid 1 grain/day.

4. We have a patient with essential hypertension who recently presented with symptoms of toxic psychosis, loss of memory, depression and agitation. She has received methyldopa 1 g/day for $4\frac{1}{2}$ weeks. Are these symptoms drug-induced?

5. Cite a recent article that reports thyrotoxicosis from cyclophosphamide therapy.

6. You know that C. March and others have studied the effects of topical flurandrenolone on adrenal function and their results appeared sometime in 1965. In which journal did this article appear?

7. A physician calls requesting information on the possibility of monilial septicemia from hyperalimentation. Cite one article.

8. Phenylbutazone has been reported to cause chromosomal damage. Document this statement with two articles.

9. Where could you find the use of a new investigational drug from Mexico called Ekilid®?

10. Where can you find abstracts of the literature regarding drug abuse?

11. Where can you obtain F.I. 6654 (manufacturer)?

12. You know that sometime in 1965 Siddall reported on his studies of the toxic effects of chlorpromazine on the eye. Cite the article.

13. Thioridazine has been reported to cause ventricular arrhythmias. Document this with one article.

14. List any references concerning the use of metronidazole in amebiasis in the Cumulated 1974 *Index Medicus*.

15. Where would you begin searching for drugs reported to cause jaundice?

5

How to Evaluate
Information Sources

Behavioral Objectives For Chapter Five
How To Evaluate Information Sources

OBJECTIVE	CRITERIA FOR MEETING OBJECTIVE	SELF EVALUATION QUESTION NUMBER

The student should be able to:

5.1 Understand the importance of the pharmacist being able to evaluate drug literature	5.1.1 Discuss the rationale for a pharmacist being able to evaluate literature	5.1
5.2 Recognize the limitations of general and secondary references	5.2.1 For each type of reference source, describe the following: 5.2.11 Time obsolescence factor 5.2.12 Authors 5.2.13 References or bibliography 5.2.14 Footnoting 5.2.15 Type of available information or scope of coverage 5.2.16 Accessibility and use of information 5.2.17 Edition or updating frequency	5.2 5.4 5.5
5.3 Demonstrate an ability to evaluate primary literature	5.3.1 Develop skills to evaluate study design 5.3.11 Purpose of study 5.3.12 Methods and experimental design 5.3.13 Reported results and validity of conclusions 5.3.14 Appropriateness of statistical methods	5.3 5.4 5.5

General Discussion

An integral part of the systematic search is the ability to evaluate the literature. Literature evaluation has three aspects: (1) general reference and textbook evaluation, (2) specialized indexing abstracting sources and (3) original scientific article or literature evaluation.

The ability of the pharmacist to evaluate the various literature sources is an important and necessary skill. It requires little or no expertise to parrot information from sources without any thought, or consideration for the accuracy or inaccuracy of the information and facts written by other individuals. The simple *dispensing* of drug information is not a function that a pharmacist should always provide, and such a simplistic approach can be a professional disservice with the potential for medical-legal repercussions. However, with prudent judgment and appropriate application of the necessary skills, the pharmacist can and should provide information that he has analyzed and judged to be objective and accurate. An in-depth discussion of the topic of literature evaluation is beyond the scope of this section, which is intended as an overview, and would indeed be redundant in view of the excellent articles on the topic already available (consult Background Reading). However, the application of these concepts is an important aspect of providing drug information and the student is instructed to study the "Background Reading" references suggested at the end of this chapter before proceeding.

General References

This category of information sources is probably the one most frequently used by the majority of practicing pharmacists. Individuals who practice in a clinical setting and rely on drug literature heavily usually have a good understanding of what information is available in commonly used drug reference texts, and of the limitations of the information that is provided. The student should seek to develop this skill, with consideration of the following points.

General reference textbooks can provide easy and convenient access to the majority of drug information requests a pharmacist may encounter. A broad information background on the drug subject in question is often available and a number of texts also provide adequate in-depth discussions of specific areas of drug information. However, while many drug-related questions may be answered from a general reference, the answer provided from a general reference alone may not necessarily be totally accurate or complete. Therefore, the pharmacist should be cognizant of certain limitations of the general reference.

1. Information available in general references will not acknowledge any recent developments in the drug literature during and after the time the publication went to press.

This "time-obsolescence" factor for general references represents a major limitation that pharmacists must be aware of and must consider. To allow for this deficiency, the pharmacist should utilize other sources, such as indexing and abstracting systems, as well as the primary literature, to ensure that any additional, more up-to-date information has been located and reviewed.

2. Information available in general references represents the interpretation and presentation of the author(s).

The possibility of human error in the interpretation of the data on which the drug-related information is based is always present. In addition, the author(s), with or without accurate interpretation, may not be aware of all of the available literature and may make erroneous statements based on the omission of data. To accommodate for this deficiency, the pharmacist must often (1) refer to the reference citation or footnote cited by an author for the specific statement and then (2) review the original reference work. On this basis, the pharmacist should be able to draw a conclusion as to the validity and accuracy of the information. This technique will give the pharmacist a better understanding of the information and will enable him/her to provide a more useful answer or response. As an additional point, the pharmacist should be cautious about providing information from a general reference based on a statement that is not footnoted. Statements from general references that are not footnoted or referenced cannot be verified for their accuracy. From a pharmacist's viewpoint, such information should be considered of limited value, other than as a citation or quote directly out of that general reference.

From the preceding discussion, it should be evident that the responsibility of the pharmacist is (1) to be aware of the limitations associated with using a general reference as a source of drug information and (2) to compensate for these limitations by examining an author's statement critically and by comparing the validity of the author's statement to the original source of the author's information (i.e., reference citation or footnote), with due consideration of any new developments pertaining to the subject. This latter point may require the review of secondary and primary reference sources. Failure to make these considerations means that the pharmacist is vulnerable to providing incomplete and inaccurate drug information.

Guidelines to Evaluating General Reference Sources

The following guidelines provide a quick reference to the considerations a pharmacist should make when evaluating and utilizing information from general references.

1. Who is (are) the author(s) and what is (are) his/her (their) credentials?

Although it is not always a good generalization to assess the validity of information on the sole criteria of an author's reputation (e.g., Linus Pauling and the vitamin C issue), the fact that an author is associated with a university teaching or medical center may indicate that the author may be more diligent in assuring the accuracy and completeness of the information, and more aware of current trends and developments in the field of study. However, this may or may not be true.

2. In what year (month, where applicable) was the reference published?

Inherent to the process of publication is the time lag that exists between the writing and publishing of general references. The time lag may be as great as two to three years for books and one to two years for review articles. This therefore represents a gap in the reference's coverage of new developments and current information.

3. What edition is the reference? Is it the most current edition?

Many general references are updated periodically, usually every two to four years although some volumes are updated annually. Updated or new editions will usually incorporate new developments and information. However, it is also important to note that the most current edition may not contain all of the specific information included in previous editions. For example, the fifth edition of Goodman, L.S. and Gilman, A., *The Pharmacological Basis of Therapeutics*, does not mention that tolerance develops to the orthostatic hypotension effects of chlorpromazine, whereas the third edition does.

4. Is there a bibliography or reference list?

If so, does it appear up to date or current? What types of literature sources are quoted? (i.e., primary vs. general references)

5. Are important statements, facts, data, etc., accurately footnoted and/or referenced?

In many instances, statements that are unreferenced are of minimal value, since their accuracy or validity cannot be confirmed. A statement that is footnoted can easily be compared for accuracy and validity to the information in its reference citation. It is not unusual to find that statements made by one author do not correlate with the data that another author cited or based his/her statements on. It is also not totally unknown to find that an author has referenced a statement with an article that is unrelated to that statement (Ingelfinger, 1976).

6. What type(s) of information is (are) available from this reference, i.e., what is the reference useful for?

See Chapter Four.

7. Is the information readily available, i.e., is there easy access to the information?

Easy access to the required information is often an important factor. Time is sometimes limited and references that expedite the location of information are very useful. For example, when a pharmacist receives a question about a poisoning, an answer can be found in a text like *Clinical Toxicology of Commercial Products*, but this requires the pharmacist to read a considerable amount of written data in order to determine the agent's toxicity and its appropriate treatment. Alternatively, the pharmacist may use an information source such as *POISINDEX*, which presents information in a format that enables the pharmacist to determine toxicity and treatment information quickly.

Secondary References

As discussed in Chapter Four, secondary references represent a valuable tool for quick and selective screening of the primary literature for specific information, data, citations and articles. In some cases, these sources provide sufficient information to serve as a reference for answering drug information requests. However, secondary reference sources also have limitations which should be kept in mind.

Most secondary references represent systems which regularly review a select segment of the primary literature. Based on this presumption, the following points regarding these sources should be considered.

1. Secondary references which are primarily indexing systems (e.g., *Index Medicus, Toxicity Bibliography, Adverse Reaction Titles*) review or cover a finite number of journals.

Utilizing only one indexing system to screen and review the primary literature may result in the error of omission. Articles in journals not covered by the system will not be reviewed or indexed and therefore will not be brought to the attention of the pharmacist. This point also applies to nonindexing systems, such as the *Iowa Drug Information System, International Pharmaceutical Abstracts* and the de Haen System, which cover even fewer journals.

2. All secondary references are subject to the time lag inherent to all publications.

Although the lag time is considerably shorter than with general references (usually months instead of years; see Table I, Chapter Four), there exists the possibility that the most current literature is not covered. One mechanism to minimize this limitation is the use of *Current Contents-Clinical Practice/Life Science* or *InPharma.* These systems have even shorter lag times.

3. Secondary sources which have formats based on abstracts (e.g., *de Haen, International Pharmaceutical Abstracts, InPharma*) usually describe only articles and clinical studies from journals.

It is important to remember that most journals provide a reader correspondence forum, i.e., Letters to the Editor. Frequently, readers respond to, criticize and add new information to published articles and studies through letters. Many abstracting systems do not include this type of information and, as a result, the pharmacist using these systems may occasionally overlook important pieces of information. Systems such as *Index Medicus, de Haen Drugs in Use* or *Iowa Drug Information System* generally do include pertinent "Letters to the Editor" within the scope of their coverage.

Primary Literature

This discussion is designed to review concepts essential to the evaluation of the primary literature, with emphasis on the clinical drug trial. The primary literature contains the most recent information about drugs and, ideally, should always be used to answer in-depth inquiries about drugs, particularly for patient-related questions. The pharmacist must be able to evaluate the validity of the information he/she provides, in order for the response to be meaningful as well as accurate.

It is important to realize that the publication of an article in a respectable journal by no means assures that its contents are accurate, or that the conclusions should be hailed without justification. Ross, 1951, analyzed 100 articles which described a procedure or type of therapy in order to determine the basis upon which conclusions had been drawn. In 45 percent of the studies, the investigation established no basis for comparison (i.e., untreated control group) and the use of controls was considered inadequate in another 18 percent. Schor and Karten, 1966, evaluated 149 analytical studies and 146 case studies (or descriptions) from ten of the "most frequently read" medical journals over a period of three months. These articles were evaluated on the validity of their conclusions, based upon the design of the experiment, the type of analysis performed and the applicability of the statistical tests used or not used. Of the 149 analytical studies evaluated by this method, less than 28 percent were considered acceptable; that is, the rest of the studies' conclusions were drawn without adequate justification. Of the 146 case studies, more than 20 percent were considered unacceptable. None of the ten journals had more than a 40 percent acceptability of analytical studies; two of the ten had *no* acceptable reports. Many other investigators have also described the inadequacies inherent in the published literature (consult Background Reading List). Thus it becomes imperative that pharmacists address themselves to these inadequacies and learn to recognize a poorly designed study or an invalid conclusion.

An adequate understanding of the *fundamental purpose* of a clinical trial is required, in order to enable the student to evaluate the primary literature. As discussed by Smith and Melmon, the purpose of the clinical trial is the *evaluation* of the efficacy and toxicity of drugs in man, utilizing the scientific or experimental approach for the purpose of determining *comparative* findings from which *inferences* can be made, i.e., that the experimental findings may be generalized to future patients. The strength of the inference, i.e., how accurate and reliable the conclusions are, depends on the validity of the comparison. In turn, the comparison's validity depends on the accuracy and appropriateness of the measurements made in the study. This, of course, also requires the elimination of bias influences.

Research articles appearing in "clinically significant" medical journals usually follow a common format. Schmidt, 1975, quoting the words of A. Kohn, approached the subject of format in a tongue-in-cheek manner. However, his facetious statements probably hold some truth and the student should also be aware that familiarity with the format of scientific reports and with its limitations will facilitate his/her ability to evaluate an article. Also, for those who aspire to be authors, a knowledge of this format will be invaluable.

Format for Scientific Communication

The following section headings frequently appear in scientific reports and are generally agreed to be indicative of a standard format. The purpose of this format is to organize and communicate scientific information effectively.

Introduction. The primary purpose of the introduction is to state clearly what the experiment or clinical trial is about, i.e., to provide a statement of the specific objective of the study. Often a brief review or discussion of previous literature published on the subject may be included.

Methodology or Methods. This section usually describes the policies and procedures undertaken by the study. It usually includes, but is not necessarily limited to: a description of the patient population/sample; control methods; therapeutic parameters to be measured; laboratory methods and techniques; and statistical methods.

Results. This section presents or reports the data found from the trial and may also be supplemented by presentations in tabular and/or graphic format.

Conclusions. This section presents the author's conclusions, based on the evaluated data. Conclusions should be based on valid inferences, although this may not always be true. This section may also be called "Discussion" or "Comments." Alternatively, the discussion section may appear separately. In either case, an interpretation of the clinical significance or importance of the findings, the conclusions and the outcome of the trial are usually given.

Summary. The summary briefly presents the purpose, objectives, results and conclusions of the paper.

References. This is a listing of the sources of the citations footnoted in the paper.

Not all of the literature the student will read and evaluate will strictly follow this format. Numerous articles review the literature and provide information based on the consensus of a number of primary literature or original articles on specific clinical trials. As discussed under General References, review articles must be scrutinized closely by the pharmacist, since errors in the literature are easily perpetuated by authors of reviews who misinterpret or misquote another author's data or information. As a result, and without regard to the nature of the article, i.e., clinical trial or review article, the pharmacist should always closely examine the article for (1) accuracy of statements (2) adequate documentation of statements and (3) accurate interpretation of the articles or information or data being referred to. In most cases, this requires the pharmacist to read the original references cited (Ingelfinger, 1976).

Judging a Clinical Study

Although a detailed discussion of literature evaluation techniques is beyond the scope of this book, the student should be aware of the fundamental features of the clinical trial upon which objective evaluation can be made. The following considerations will be helpful in assessing the usefulness of a given reference article.

General Considerations

1. Is the journal in which the article appears considered to be reputable?
The more widely read medical journals generally publish better designed clinical studies. This is usually the basis for their reputation. Some of these include, but are not necessarily limited to, *American Journal of Medicine, Annals of Internal Medicine, Circulation,*

New England Journal of Medicine, Clinical Pharmacology and Therapeutics and *Mayo Clinic Proceedings* (Allyn, 1975).

2. Is the title consistent with the scope of the 'Summary'? Titles may be misleading and the reader should never make claims about a study based on its title alone. By referring to the summary of the paper, one can ascertain if the title is indeed erroneous. Including the terms "double blind," "randomized," or "crossover" in the title does not necessarily mean the study is valid. Titles may be useful to determine if a study is applicable to a particular situation or drug problem.

3. Are the investigators considered to be reliable and was the study conducted in a reputable medical center or university teaching hospital? If not, is the location adequate for the application of good scientific experimental methods? In general, the better clinical studies are performed by clinical pharmacologists and/or specialists within the given field. This is important, as it means that the investigators are familiar with the drug and disease state in question, as well as with the fundamentals of experimental design. In addition, most clinical pharmacologists and specialists have access to a large medical center and facilities which enable adequate population samples with control groups to be established, together with adequate follow-through of the study design.

Specific Considerations

1. Are the objectives and/or hypotheses (i.e., purpose) of the study well-defined? The objectives of the study should be clearly stated and the investigator should define the response he is looking for to indicate the safety or efficacy of the drug. Ideally, all areas of subjectivity and bias on the part of the investigator should be absent or negated in the study. However, in most cases the author desires proof of the drug's effectiveness and may have preconceived notions about the study's results. Occasionally, this enthusiasm enters the study objectives and may create a pattern throughout the trial. For example, an investigator may state: "The objective of the present study is to evaluate the effectiveness of dipyridamole, an effective coronary vasodilator, in the management and prophylaxis of acute episodes of angina pectoris." This statement implies bias and could be construed to mean that improvement in coronary blood flow will be beneficial to angina patients. For this particular example, the reader must analyze this statement, and the data in the study, with the following questions in mind: "Does increased coronary blood flow equate with improved flow to ischemic areas?" "Does coronary vasodilation in fact signify an increase in coronary blood flow?" "What parameters is the author using as an index of improvement in coronary vessel dilation?" "If 80 out of 100 patients improve on the drug, is this a placebo effect or a result of improved coronary blood flow?" (Walton, 1972)

Smith and Melmon (1978) emphasize asking the following questions when evaluating the objectives of a clinical trial.

  a. Is there a well-defined (simple) objective? Has a question or hypothesis been stated clearly?

  b. Has the author defined the response which is to be indicative of efficacy or safety?

  c. Do you understand what the author considers to be clinically important or meaningful? Do you agree?

2. Were appropriate scientific methods and experimental design employed for this type of study?

  a. How large was the population sample? Was the population sample described adequately? Were the subjects chosen by appropriate means?

A large population sample is of course desired, but is not always possible. However, the number of patients in the study should be representative of the problem under study if the results are to be extrapolated. For case studies, one or two patients may be acceptable if the description of the case is significantly detailed to be meaningful. Case studies are of value, especially if the disease state or condition is rarely encountered and there are insufficient numbers of patients to conduct suitable clinical trials. A case study of carbamazepine (Tegretol®) in hemifacial spasms may be significant if the author describes the case adequately and provides meaningful follow-up. Adverse reaction case reports may also be considered significant if a definite cause-effect relationship has been established. However, for the clinical trial, a sufficient patient sample should be included for statistical analysis to reveal any significant difference between the drug and control groups. The number of patients in a trial is a good indication of the scope and validity of the study and, as a general rule for well-designed studies, the larger the population sample the more useful the results.

Since the goal of a clinical trial is to be able to extrapolate the findings to future patients, i.e., make inferences, the investigator must provide a detailed description of the patient population admitted to the study. This will enable the reader to make inferences about the types of patients the results may be applicable to.

In the absence of an adequate description of the population

sample or criteria for admission to the study, there is no basis upon which inferences can be made. Sorby defines "general population" as all individuals on whom a drug might eventually be used, and stresses the importance of the investigator selecting the sample of test subjects on the basis of the population being studied. The results of the study will therefore indicate how the drug will act in that specific population. It is obvious that if there is an inadequate description of the general population (types of subjects under study), the reader will not know what types of patients the results actually apply to.

Examples of descriptions of general populations might be:

Oral Hypoglycemic agent. Adult onset diabetics with a blood sugar of 130–150 mg%.

Diazoxide. All patients with malignant hypertension due to renal disease.

Nitroprusside Sodium. All patients with malignant hypertension (diastolic of 140–180 mm Hg).

Propoxyphene. Females (24–36 years of age) with episiotomy pain.

Haloperidol. Patients with undifferentiated, chronic schizophrenia unresponsive to phenothiazines.

It is also important that the investigator insure that the test subjects *represent* the general population; that is, all of the variables and idiosyncrasies found in the general population should also be present in the test subjects. These include age, sex, weight, genetic background and severity of disease state. No matter how well the general population is defined, not all patients will respond in exactly the same way, and the test group should preferably not contain any unusual variables not found in the general population. This is also referred to as a "homogeneous" patient population, meaning that within the test group all subjects are equally likely, before treatment, to respond to the drug under study. Populations that do not adhere to this description are called "heterogeneous."

A homogeneous population that is a fully representative sample of patients may be selected by employing a *randomized* selection process i.e., "random sampling." The selection of test subjects from the total group of available subjects is made entirely by chance and is therefore not subject to sampling bias on the part of the investigator. Thus, every subject has an equal and independent chance of being included in a sample (Saiger, 1960).

It is important to note that since the composition of a random sample will vary, the sample may not be characteristic of the population which it is chosen to represent. However, it does provide the primary means for gauging the validity of the inferences that can be made from the study results.

Examples of sampling bias include:

Stratified sample. Subjects admitted on basis of sex (i.e., female, male) alone, without selecting members of various categories at random.

Volunteer Sample. Subjects admitted to a study on a voluntary basis.

Selection. Subjects admitted on the basis of certain factors such as health habits or on the basis of interviewers selecting the subjects.

b. Were adequate methods and experimental design used to insure that the results obtained were valid and free from bias?

Was the trial prospective or retrospective? A prospective design permits advance planning to study experimental groups before the group is exposed to the drug or therapeutic manipulation. This type of trial permits the investigator to establish better methods for controls, randomization and data collection. Retrospective trials refer to research done *after* the population has been treated with the drug. In this type of study researchers must collect data, usually by means of chart reviews. These data, which are documented (or omitted) by multiple observers in the charts, may often be subject to hidden and/or overt biases, as well as arbitrary drug treatment allocations (Weitzman, 1974).

Were adequate controls established? A study should establish a basis for the comparative evaluation of the drug under identical conditions and include controls, usually by establishing a treatment group and a control group. Control groups should be comparable to the treatment group except for the factor being tested, i.e., new drug treatment vs. control treatment (e.g., treatment with another, similar, accepted drug). Controls should also be concurrent in time and place with respect to the subjects receiving the treatment. This is necessary if unbiased comparisons between current and previous data and experiences are desired. If the test and control groups are not comparable, any differences noted may be due to the lack of comparability rather than to the new drug treatment. For example, trials not concurrent in time may be subject to biases from general advances in medical care.

In certain clinical situations controls may be unnecessary, such as in the treatment of a disease which is universally or rapidly fatal. Since a suitable basis for comparison already exists, any improvement in survival rate will have been the result of the new drug treatment. In this circumstance, a "historical control," i.e., previous high mortality rate, is utilized.

In serious disease states, e.g., pseudomonas infections, new drug treatment is compared against controls using currently approved or standard methods of drug therapy, e.g., gentamicin vs. a new aminoglycoside. For less serious illnesses or where only symptoms of disease processes (e.g., pain, urticaria) are treated, a new drug's therapeutic benefits must be compared to a placebo preparation as well as to any current standard of therapy. The placebo is a preparation intended to endow the psychological influence of drug treatment to a subject without any pharmacologic effect.

In some clinical situations, a subject or patient may serve as his own control, e.g., as in studies of drugs in chronic diseases or where subjects are given different drug treatments in sequence or in an alternating manner. This latter method is usually referred to as "crossover." However, crossover methods do not necessarily add to the validity of the trial unless the duration of drug treatment before crossover accounts for the time of onset of the drug's therapeutic effect. This is particularly important if the drug's onset of action is very long. Similarly, following the crossover, the duration of a drug's effect after its discontinuation must be considered when observing and recording results data.

Were drug and control treatments allocated to the subjects in a random manner? The allocation of treatment to the subjects must be based upon a random selection method. This is to assure that the trial is free from any unconscious selection bias that the investigator may introduce, such as preconceived opinions, which may affect treatment allocation. The random allocation of treatment may be accomplished by tossing a coin or by utilizing a table of random numbers found in statistical texts.

Where prior knowledge of the disease state may influence the outcome, patients may be grouped or stratified together using separate randomization series for these groups. This results in a more uniform distribution of patients within different subgroups and the various treatments will then be administered to representative samples of the total patient series being studied.

Without random allocation, bias, either deliberate or unconscious, may influence treatment allocation and prevent each subject from having an equal chance of receiving the new drug treatment. In addition, there is no established guarantee for the balance of treatment groups for unknown variables and for the validity of the statistical tests of significance used to compare the treatments (Mahon, 1964; Bryar, 1976).

Were adequate blinding techniques utilized? The use of blinding techniques is most important in the evaluation of the results of new drug treatments, when the effect of drugs on subjective responses is measured and the potential for the introduction of bias into the study results exists. In double-blind studies, neither the subject nor the observing investigator is aware of the allocation of the new drug treatment. When improvement in symptoms or general clinical appearance are the measurable parameters, a double-blind design prevents the hopes and prejudices of the observers or investigators from influencing the conclusions. The single blind technique only renders the patient unaware of whether he/she is receiving a placebo or active drug.

Were appropriate considerations for the proper use of the drug made? To assess a drug's therapeutic merit properly, it must be used appropriately. Factors which may influence the drug's therapeutic and toxic effects must be considered and accounted for in the study. The following points should therefore be evaluated.

(1) Were drug doses and regimens within the therapeutic range?

An inappropriate dose may result in the inaccurate or misleading evaluation of a drug. A suboptimal dose may result in no or subtherapeutic effects, whereas an excessive dose may result in excessive side effects or toxic manifestations. Similarly, the dosage interval (i.e., times of administration) or route of administration may have some bearing on drug effects. Bioavailability differences between different routes of administration must also be considered.

(2) Was the duration of the trial adequate?

This factor should be considered, with an emphasis on the time required for the onset of optimal drug effects. If a drug's effects do not become apparent until after two to four weeks of continuous administration, e.g., as with the tricyclic antidepressants, the trial must be at least four weeks long and preferably longer. Similarly, for crossover trial designs, discontinuation of the drug treatment and switching to a placebo or other treatment must account for the time for the first drug's effect to dissipate.

(3) Were any drugs used concurrently, and if so were they accounted for?

Concomitant drug administration may influence the results of a trial and must therefore be accounted for. Drug interactions may be possible and this risk is ever present.

Were appropriate considerations made for the correct measurement of the established parameters of therapeutic efficacy? The following criteria should be evaluated:

(1) Number and type of observers;

(2) Methods of collection:

Were the measureable parameters indicative of therapeutic effectiveness?

Are factors known which may influence the parameters measured?

What are the characteristics of the test methods used to assess these parameters and what factors may influence the accuracy of the test methods?

Were standard measurements used and are they reproducible?

Were the results reported accurately? The investigator should mention all aspects pertinent to the results of the trial. Omission of data or the failure to describe certain data adequately may leave doubt in one's mind as to the report's accuracy or validity. The following points are often important:

Were side effects reported, including the nature and incidence of the reactions?

Were dropouts reported and the precise reasons for their dismissal given?

Were there any missing or unreconcilable data?

Were appropriate statistical methods utilized?

Were valid conclusions drawn, i.e., were the conclusions of the study actually supported by the results? The pharmacist must distinguish between biased impressions and inferences based on valid comparisons. In addition, extrapolation of data and conclusions beyond the conditions of the study must be avoided. It is important to note that even though in many studies the conclusions can be made readily, occasionally some investigators may draw distorted conclusions from their results. Conclusions must also be placed in their proper clinical perspective; the pharmacist should consider the effectiveness and toxicity of the drug under study *compared to* other similar therapeutic agents presently on the market. For example, demonstrating that a new phenothiazine is equivalent to, or more effective than, haloperidol for acute screaming episodes is important, but is the new phenothiazine *better* than other available phenothiazines for this indication?

Does the article provide a reference list or bibliography to verify footnoted citations? The judicious use of footnoting and references often provides support and validity to the information found in the article. In fact, the absence of this information prevents the reader from obtaining additional data, as well as from verifying the article's credibility. However, the mere presence of footnoting and references in an article does not necessarily guarantee its validity. Primary or other sources cited may have been "misquoted, inapplicable, unreliable and occasionally even imaginary" (Ingelfinger, 1976).

Appropriateness of Statistical Methods

Although a detailed and comprehensive discussion of statistical analysis and evaluation techniques is beyond the scope of this book, the student should be aware of some of the more basic and fundamental features of statistics. The following considerations will be helpful in evaluating primary literature. First, however, a brief annotated glossary is presented, in order to acquaint the student or practitioner with the terminology he is likely to encounter in a presentation or discussion of statistics or the results of statistical analyses.

Annotated Glossary of Terms

Population and sample, parameter and statistic.
A population is a group which contains every member that fits the description of the population. For example, the population of "hospital patients" includes all patients who are currently in a hospital, as well as all who have ever been in a hospital and all who will ever be in a hospital. A description of that group (average blood pressure, variability of performance on some manual dexterity task, etc.) is called a parameter. Whenever parameters are available, no tests for significance or any other inferential procedures are necessary, because all possible members of the group are included in the calculation of the parameter.

It is probably evident to the student that there are very few situations in which parameters are available, the exceptions being populations which are so restricted as to be of little general interest. For example, a population could be defined as "all patients in hospital X during July, 1978," but most researchers are interested in generalizing beyond that limited group. Generalization is legitimate if that group is considered one of many possible samples of all hospitalized patients. Samples are selected in situations where the population of interest is not available, or is so large that parameters cannot be obtained without tremendous expense. A selected sample is used to estimate the population parameters, and it is here that statistics (the sample equivalents of parameters) and statistical inference come into play.

Measures of central tendency
Mean (Arithmetic Mean). The mean is often denoted as $\overline{X}$ or M and is the same as what is commonly called the average. It is

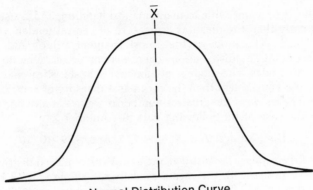

Normal Distribution Curve

Normal curve: If infinite samples of a population are drawn, the subjects' scores on a selected parameter will be normally distributed

Figure 1

obtained by adding up all the individual values and dividing by the total number of items. The mean is the most frequently used measure of central tendency (Figure 1). It is also the most commonly used statistical average and is highly amenable to statistical manipulation. Thus:

$$\bar{X} = \frac{1}{n} \sum_{i=1}^{n} x_i$$

Where,

$\sum$ = sigma (symbol for summation)
x_i = individual values of observations being summed
n = total number of observations

If individual values for six observations are 1, 3, 5, 7, 9, 11, the mean is:

$$\bar{X} = \frac{1}{6}(1 + 3 + 5 + 7 + 9 + 11) = \frac{36}{6} = 6$$

Median. The median is defined as the "middle value" of a set of ordered data. It is often useful because it is not sensitive to occasional extreme values. For example, the median of the data set: 1, 2, 3, 4, 5 is 3; the median of the set: 1, 2, 3, 4, 5000 is still 3, although the means of the two groups are very different. The median is often thought of as the "most typical" value; for example, the government reports median (not mean) incomes. However, the median is less amenable to mathematical handling and is used less frequently than the mean as a measure of central tendency.

Mode. The mode is the "most frequent value" and is the highest point of a distribution. There may on occasion be no mode or many modes. The mode is not amenable to statistical manipulations and is used less than the mean as a measure of central tendency. The mode is the greatest number of values at any one point, or in the case of the following data, the number 7.

Data Values: 2, 5, 5, 6, 7, 7, 7, 8, 8, 9, 9, 10, 10

Relationship to the Distribution Curve. With a normal distribution curve (symmetrical), the mean, median and mode will all be the same (Figure 2A). In a skewed distribution curve, the median will lie between the mean and the mode (Figure 2B). When the fre-

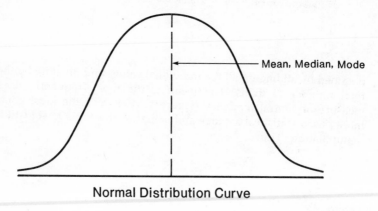

Normal Distribution Curve

Figure 2A

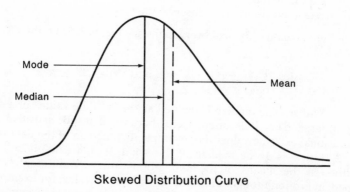

Skewed Distribution Curve

Figure 2B

quency distribution is skewed to the right (positive), as in Figure 2B, the mean is to the right of the mode.

Measures of Variability

The most commonly used measures of variability are the variance, symbolized by s^2, and its square root, the standard deviation, signified by S or SD. Both are used to describe the degree of dispersion of individual values from the mean. They measure the average spread of all points from the mean. Standard deviation from the mean is the quadratic mean (or root mean square) of the derivations from the arithmetic mean; that is, the values that may be expected to occur above and below the mean ($\overline{X}$). Figure 3 presents standard deviations for a normal distribution curve.

For a normal curve, about 68 percent of the values in the population will lie in the range from $\overline{X} - S$ to $\overline{X} + S$ (Mean value plus or minus one standard deviation). Similarly, about 96 percent of all values in the population will lie within $\overline{X} - 2S$ to $\overline{X} + 2S$. Virtually all values (i.e., 99.5 percent) in the population will lie within $\overline{X} \pm 3S$ (see Figure 3).

Statistical Inference

Knowing something about the nature of the sample obtained in a scientific study enables the researcher to make some inferences

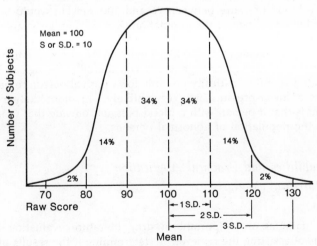

Standard deviations from the mean

Figure 3

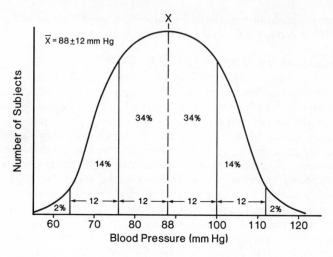

Figure 4

about the population from which the sample was drawn. This principle is frequently used in clinical settings as a guide to diagnosis. Let us examine a particular situation and see how statistics can be (and are) routinely applied.

If the mean diastolic blood pressure in a normal adult population sample is 88 mm Hg, and the standard deviation is 12 mm Hg, then a blood pressure between 76 and 100 mm Hg would be expected in 68 percent of the population ($\bar{X} \pm S$). Similarly, about 96 percent of the population would have blood pressures in the range of 64 to 112 mm Hg ($\bar{X} \pm 2S$) (See Figure 4). Any pressure higher or lower than those values is generally considered pathological. Even though it is still statistically possible for a normal person to have a higher or lower pressure, it is very unlikely. The more likely explanation is that a person with a blood pressure outside that range is from the population of abnormal persons.

Probabilities and Practical Application of Statistical Analysis

Statistics are important in drug literature evaluation as a means of assisting the reviewer in determining if the results of the study have been legitimately extrapolated to the general population, i.e., whether proper inferences have been made. Statistical procedures utilize the aforementioned parameters to determine the probability of making an error when extrapolating sets of data.

Probability is an important facet of statistical analysis. For example, if a coin is flipped ten times, there is a given probability that the coin will turn up heads a certain percentage of the time and tails a certain percentage of the time. Specifically, the likelihood of flipping a coin ten times and getting five heads and five tails is 0.667, or the likelihood of six tails and four heads is 0.205. On the other hand, the probability of getting all heads or all tails is only 0.001. Therefore, statistical inferences represent a question of probabilities; that is, given the results obtained, how probable are the results? Are the results a likely occurrence or an unlikely occurrence without the treatment?

These same methods are employed in clinical studies. Probability values are determined to decide if the results obtained are due to actual effects or to chance. In virtually every clinical study, the investigator makes the prior assumption that there is no effect, e.g., no significant difference between the means of the two test groups. This is referred to as the "null hypothesis." He then sets out to determine the likelihood that the null hypothesis is right or wrong.

In this kind of inferential situation, four different outcomes are possible. The experimenter may correctly infer that his experiment resulted in no effect, if indeed there was no effect, or he may correctly detect an effect that was present. The remaining two outcomes result in an incorrect decision: the conclusion that an effect exists when in fact none does (Type I error), and the conclusion that there was no effect when one was present (Type II error) (see Figure 5).

Type I error is generally regarded as more serious than Type II error and consequently more precautions are taken to minimize the risks of incurring such an error. This is accomplished by requiring that the result obtained be sufficiently different from the result expected under the null hypothesis (the hypothesis of "no effect"),

		The "Truth"	
		No Effect	Effect
Inference Based on Experimental Results	Effect	Incorrect: Type I Error	Correct Effect Exists
	No Effect	Correct: No Effect	Incorrect: Type II Error

Figure 5. Inferential Outcomes of Experimental Results

such that the inference of chance alone being responsible for the effect is very unlikely. The allowable likelihood of a Type I error is expressed as a "P" value.

"P" refers to the probability that the reader is wrong in rejecting the null hypothesis. A 95 percent confidence interval is usually used to represent validity of results; that is, the investigator attempts to prove that the results obtained in his group of patients are correct and not due to chance for more than 95 percent of the time. Thus, a P value of 0.05 indicates that there is a 5 percent chance the reader is wrong in rejecting the null hypothesis, i.e., in saying that there is an effect when there is none. If P is less than 0.05 ($P < 0.05$), there is less than a 5 percent chance that the reader is wrong in rejecting the null hypothesis and the results are considered statistically significant (i.e., there is less than a 5 percent chance that they are due to chance alone).

Some examples of probability values presented in the literature and their significance are presented below.

$P \leq 0.001$. If a P value of less than 0.001 is reported, then the means ($\overline{X}$) of the treatment and control groups are significantly different and there is less than a 0.1 percent chance that they may really not be different (i.e., the null hypothesis is rejected) or that the effects are due to chance alone.

$P < 0.15$. If a P value of less than 0.15 is reported, then the means are not significantly different (at the 95 percent interval) and the null hypothesis is not rejected, i.e., there is no effect. If the reader rejects the null hypothesis, it indicates the difference of the means is significant with a 15 percent chance of error. In most studies, this P value is considered unacceptable.

$0.10 > P > 0.05$. When P values are stated in this manner, the probability of incorrectly rejecting the null hypothesis lies between 5 percent and 10 percent.

Summary

Statistics are frequently used in research for describing data and making inferences about sets of data. Although a statistically significant difference does not necessarily validate a study or the clinical significance of that study's finding, a basic understanding of this information is mandatory in order for the pharmacist to evaluate the results of clinical drug trials.

Table 1. Evaluation of Primary Literature Checklist

ITEM	EVALUATION DISCUSSED?	YES/NO

General Considerations of the Study

1. Is the journal in which the article appears considered to be a reputable one? _____ _____
2. Is the title consistent with the scope of the "summary"? _____ _____
3. Are the investigators considered to be reliable and was the study conducted in a reputable medical center or university teaching hospital? If not, is the location adequate for the application of good scientific experimental methods? _____ _____

Specific Considerations of the Study

1. Are the objectives and/or hypothesis (i.e., purpose) of the study well-defined? _____ _____
2. Were appropriate scientific methods of experimental design employed for this type of study? _____ _____
   a. How large was the population sample? Was the population sample described adequately? Were the subjects chosen by appropriate means? _____ _____
   b. Were adequate methods and experimental design used to insure that the results obtained were valid and free from bias? _____ _____
      (1) Was the trial prospective or retrospective? _____ _____
      (2) Were adequate controls established? _____ _____
      (3) Were drug and control treatments allocated to the subjects in a random manner? _____ _____
      (4) Were adequate blinding techniques utilized? _____ _____
      (5) Were appropriate considerations for the proper use of the drug made? _____ _____
         (a) Were drug doses and regimens within the therapeutic range? _____ _____
         (b) Was the duration of the trial adequate? _____ _____
         (c) Were any drugs used concurrently and if so were they accounted for? _____ _____
      (6) Were appropriate considerations made for the correct measurement of the established parameters of therapeutic efficacy? _____ _____
         (a) Number and type of observers _____ _____
         (b) Methods of collection
            i. Were the measurable parameters indicative of therapeutic effectiveness? _____ _____
            ii. Are factors known which may influence the parameters measured? _____ _____

continued

Table 1. Evaluation of Primary Literature Checklist (*continued*)

ITEM	EVALUATION DISCUSSED?	YES/NO
iii. What are the characteristics of the test methods used to assess these parameters and what factors may influence the accuracy of the test methods?	_____	_____
iv. Were standard measurements used and are they reproducible?	_____	_____
(7) Were the results reported accurately?	_____	_____
(a) Were side effects reported, including the nature and incidence of the reactions?	_____	_____
(b) Were dropouts reported and the precise reasons for their dismissal given?	_____	_____
(c) Were they any missing or unreconcilable data?	_____	_____
(d) Were appropriate statistical methods utilized?	_____	_____
(8) Were valid conclusions drawn, i.e., were the conclusions of the study actually supported by the results?	_____	_____
(9) Does the article provide a reference list or bibliography to verify footnoted citations?	_____	_____

Background Reading

Reviews

1. Allyn, R.H.: The Literature of Medicine: A Library for Internists II., *Ann.Intern.Med.* 84:346–373, 1976
2. Buncher, C.R.: Principles of Experimental Design for Clinical Drug Studies *In* Francke, D.E. and Whitney, H.A.K., Jr. (Eds.), *Perspectives in Clinical Pharmacy*, 1st Ed., Drug Intelligence Publications, Inc. Hamilton, Illinois, 1972, p. 504
3. Madden, M. and MacDonald, A.: An Evaluation and Comparison of Nine Drug Information Retrieval Services, *Drug Inform.J.*: 47–59, 1977
4. Schmidt, R.: How to Prepare a Manuscript, *N.Engl.J.Med.* 293:441, 1975
5. Smith, W., and Melmon, K.: Drug Choice in Disease *In* Melmon, K. and Morelli, H.F. (Eds.), *Clinical Pharmacology-Basic Principles in Therapeutics*, 2nd Ed., Macmillan Co., New York, N.Y., 1978
6. Sorby, D.L.: Evaluation of Drug Literature, Unpublished Report
7. Walton, C.A.: Drug Literature Utilization: Selection, Evaluation and Communication *In* Blisset et al. (Eds.), *Clinical Pharmacy Practice*, Lea and Febiger, Philadelphia, Pennsylvania, 1972, p. 349

Evaluation of General and Secondary References

1. Ascione, F.J.: Information Sources—Separating Fact from Fiction, *Drug Ther.* 1:33–39, 1976
2. Bell, J.E.: Comparative Evaluation of Drug Interaction Publications, *Am.J.Hosp.Pharm.* 33:1299–1303 (Dec.) 1976

3. Cardoni, A.A.: Comparison of Current Content's Life Sciences and Clinical Practice Edition, *Am.J.Hosp.Pharm. 30*:721-722, 1973
4. Ingelfinger, F.J.: Seduction by Citation, *N.Engl.J.Med. 295*:1074-1075, 1976
5. Tourville, J.F. and McLeod, D.C.: Comparison of the Clinical Utility of Four Drug Information Services, *Am.J.Hosp.Pharm. 32*:1153-1158, 1975

Evaluation of Primary Literature

1. Badgley, R.: An Assessment of Research Methods Reported in 103 Scientific Articles from Two Canadian Medical Journals, *Can.Med.Assoc.J. 85*:246-250, 1961
2. Byar, D.P. et al.: Randomized clinical trials, *N.Engl.J.Med. 295*:74-80, 1976
3. Feinstein, A.R.: Clinical Epidemiology: The Clinical Design of Statistics in Therapy, *Ann.Intern.Med. 69*:1287-1312, 1968
4. Gross, H. et al.: Anticoagulant therapy in Myocardial Infarction, An Overview of Methodology, *Am.J.Med. 52*:421-424, 1972
5. Gifford, R.H. and Feinstein, A.R.: A Critique of Methodology in Studies of Anticoagulant Therapy for Acute Myocardial Infarction, *N.Engl.J.Med. 280*:351-357, 1969
6. Harris, L.: Some Problems of Therapeutic Trials in Hypertension, *J.Clin.Pharmacol. 16*:165-170, 1976
7. Ingelfinger, F.J.: Seduction by Citation, *N.Engl.J.Med. 295*:1074-1075, 1976
8. Lionel, N.D.W. and Herxheimer, A.: Assessing Reports of Therapeutic Trials, *Br.Med.J. 3*:637-640, 1970
9. Mahon, W.A. et al.: A Method for the Assessment of Reports of Drug Trials, *Can.Med.Assoc.J. 90*:565, 1964
10. Mainland, D.: The Clinical Trial—Some Difficulties and Suggestions, *J.Chron.Dis. 11*:484-496, 1960
11. Mainland, D.: The Significance of "Nonsignificance," *Clin. Pharmacol.Ther. 4*:580-586, 1963
12. Modell, W., Houde, R.W.: Factors Influencing Clinical Evaluation of Drugs, *J.Am.Med.Assoc. 167*:2190-2198, 1958
13. Modell, W.: The Sensitivity and Validity of Drug Evaluations in Man, *Clin.Pharmacol.Ther. 1*:769-776, 1960
14. Nash, H.: The Double-Blind Procedure: Rationale and Empirical Evaluation, *J.Nerv.Ment.Dis. 134*:34-47, 1962
15. Rinzler, S.H.: Symposium on Clinical Drug Evaluation and Human Pharmacology, *Clin.Pharmacol.Ther. 3*:505-509, 1962
16. Ross, O.B., Jr.: Use of Controls in Medical Research, *J.Am.Med.Assoc. 145*:72, 1951
17. Saiger, G.L.: Errors of Medical Studies, *J.Am.Med.Assoc. 173*:678-681, 1960
18. Schmidt, R.N.: How to Prepare a Manuscript, *N.Engl.J.Med. 293*:411, 1975
19. Schor, S. and Karten, I.: Statistical Evaluation of Medical Journal Manuscripts, *J.Am.Med.Assoc. 195*:1123-1128, 1966
20. Weitzmen, S. and Berger, S.: Clinical Trial Design in Studies of Corticosteroids for Bacterial Infections, *Ann.Intern.Med. 81*:36-42, 1974
21. Peto, R. et al.: Design and Analysis of Randomized Clinical Trials Requiring Prolonged Observation of Each Patient I. Introduction and Design, *Br.J.Cancer 34*:585-612, 1976
22. Peto, R. et al.: Design and Analysis of Randomized Clinical Trials Requiring Prolonged Observation of Each Patient II. Analysis and Examples, *Br.J.Cancer 35*:1-39, 1977

Self Evaluation Questions and Learning Examples on How to Evaluate Information Sources

5.1 Discuss the pharmacist's need of an ability to evalute literature.

5.2 Identify seven considerations and criteria for evaluating general and secondary reference sources.

5.3 Identify the appropriate criteria for evaluating primary literature and discuss the implications of these with respect to clinical study design and their results.

5.4 *Learning Examples.* Obtain the following citations from a medical library and evaluate them on the basis of the criteria discussed in this chapter, using Table 1.

   a. Fisher, B. et al.: 1-Phenylalanine Mustard (L-Pam) in the Management of Primary Breast Cancer, *N.Engl.J.Med.* 292:117–122, 1975

   b. Gallant, D. et al.: Loxapine: A Six Month Evaluation in Severely Ill Schizophrenic Patients, *Curr.Ther.Res.* 15:205–209, 1973

   c. Report from the Boston Collaborative Drug Surveillance Program: Reserpine and Breast Cancer, *Lancet* 2:669–671, 1974

   d. Le Pere, D.: Evaluation of a New Symptomatic Treatment for Meniere's Disease, *Clin.Med.*:63–64 (Apr) 1967

   e. Litchfield, H.R. and Halperin, J.: Iron Deficiency Anemia, *Med.Times* 89:1187–1195, 1961

   f. Paris, L. and Newfield, H.: Morning Stiffness and Arthritis, *Clin.Med.* 8:2029, 1963

   g. Ferebee, S.H. et al.: The Use of Chemotherapy as a Prophylactic Measure in Tuberculosis, *Ann.N.Y.Acad.Sci.* 106:151, 1963

   h. Salzman, E.W. and Harris, W.H.: Reduction in Venous Thromboembolism by Agents Affecting Platelet Function, *N.Engl.J.Med.* 284:1287–1292, 1971

   i. McMahon, F.G.: Efficacy of an Antihypertensive Agent, *J.Am.Med.Assoc.* 231:155–158, 1975

   j. Greenstein, J.S.: Studies on a New, Peerless Contraceptive Agent: A Preliminary Final Report, *Can.Med.Assoc.J.* 93:1351–1355, 1965

5.5 *Learning Examples.* Identify the classification type and missing background and history information, then prepare a written response utilizing the recommended format for the following case examples. The key to these examples is in the "Case Histories" located in Chapter 8.

a. How effective is mithramycin in Paget's disease? How does it compare to other agents that have been used?

b. How effective is low molecular weight dextran (dextran 40) in the prevention of thromboembolism following fractures?

c. Is colchicine of any real value in the prophylaxis of acute attacks of gout? Are any toxic effects associated with long term prophylactic use?

d. What is the risk of teratogenicity with rubella vaccine? Is abortion indicated?

e. What doses of Darvon Compound®-65 are required to produce physical dependence?

f. What is the recommended dosage of betamethasone to prevent respiratory depression in the newborn?

g. How clinically significant is a methylphenidate-tricyclic antidepressant interaction?

6

How to Formulate and Communicate a Response

Behavioral Objectives For Chapter Six
How to Formulate and Communicate a Response

OBJECTIVE	CRITERIA FOR MEETING OBJECTIVE	SELF EVALUATION QUESTION NUMBER
The student should:		
6.1 Demonstrate an ability to formulate retrieved information into a suitable format for verbal or written communication	6.1.1 Develop skills in formulating a response 6.1.11 List information retrieved into a logical format 6.1.12 Summarize data into a useful form	6.1 6.5
6.2 Demonstrate the ability to prepare a written response	6.2.1 Identify essential parameters required for written response 6.2.11 Request/Background Information 6.2.12 Response: Introduction/Background Findings Tables, Graphs, Charts 6.2.13 Conclusion 6.2.14 References	6.2 6.5
6.3 Demonstrate an awareness of the skills necessary to communicate a verbal response	6.3.1 Identify specific guidelines helpful in communicating a response verbally	6.3 6.5

continued

Behavioral Objectives For Chapter Six
How to Formulate and
Communicate a Response (*continued*)

OBJECTIVE	CRITERIA FOR MEETING OBJECTIVE	SELF EVALUATION QUESTION NUMBER
6.4 Demonstrate an awareness of the importance of providing follow-up to an answer	6.4.1 Identify the reasons for providing follow-up responses 6.4.11 Correct question/ response 6.4.12 Impact of response 6.4.13 Further assistance	6.4 6.5

General Discussion

It should be obvious to the pharmacist that searching the literature comes before formulating and/or writing a response (Beatty, 1973). However, prior to even initiating an answer or response to a question or request, the pharmacist should have firmly in mind what is required for the answer. The information that has been found through research must answer the specific needs of the question and its clinical circumstances. It is very important that the pharmacist provide information that is clinically *applicable*. A second important consideration is that the pharmacist *organize* the information such that the answer is presented in a *"pharmaceutically elegant"* manner. It should be obvious that in addition to good organization, the correct rules of grammar, syntax, punctuation and spelling should always be observed.

Communication skills are critical to the provision of drug information and the pharmacist must be able to present information in a manner which will be understood by the caller. Unless the information is communicated effectively, it makes no difference how much is available or how useful it may be. Reading out of a textbook or citing one or two clinical studies may not be sufficient when providing clinically oriented drug information. The pharmacist must communicate the response in a manner which will *answer* the question and not merely provide information which pertains to it. To accomplish this, he/she must fully understand why the question is being asked, which requires a knowledge of all pertinent background data that may modify the response. Unless it is known why the question is being asked, an optimally useful, informative response cannot be supplied. These concepts have been discussed in Chapter Three, but a further discussion is warranted here.

Some questions occur without background circumstances. An example may be when a caller requests a summary of the available literature on a given subject. Examples of these types of questions are: "How effective is aspirin and dipyridamole in preventing thromboembolism?" "How effective is dantrolene sodium in multiple sclerosis patients?" "What is the current status of swine flu vaccination?" These questions may be answered by a review of the literature, a summary of the findings and an appropriate conclusion. However, the majority of drug information questions received by a pharmacist are generated by underlying circumstances. Hence, the question, "Is there any interaction between Esimil® and Zyloprim®?" could be answered in the following manner:

Esimil® contains hydrochlorothiazide 25 mg and guanethidine 10 mg per tablet. There are no significant interactions between allopurinol (Zyloprim®) and guanethidine. The hypouricemic effects of allopurinol can be antagonized by the concomitant administration of hydrochlorothiazide, but this is of questionable significance since allopurinol is used to treat thiazide-induced hyperuricemia.[1,2] However, gouty patients receiving allopurinol should be monitored closely for possible exacerbation of symptoms if Esimil® is added to the regimen.

References
1. Nicotero, J.A. et al.: Prevention of Hyperuricemia by Allopurinol in Hypertensive Patients Treated with Chlorothiazide, *N.Engl.J.Med.* 282:133, 1970
2. Rapado, A.: Allopurinol in Thiazide-Induced Hyperuricemia, *Ann.Rheum.Dis.* 25:660, 1966

However, upon questioning the physician on the circumstances or reason behind the question, the following is revealed: "We have a 51-year-old, 180 pound female who was admitted for low back pain. She has a long history of hypertension which has been controlled successfully with Esimil® 2 tabs daily and Aldomet® 250 mg daily for 2 years. She is also receiving Valium 5 mg qid. She has asymptomatic hyperuricemia of unknown etiology and her uric acid (SMA) on admission was 9.2 mg%. We've started her on Zyloprim® 100 mg tid. Is there any problem giving Zyloprim® to a patient on Esimil®? I've heard something, somewhere about that."

The additional information changes the scope of the question and it becomes a different problem to that of a simple drug interaction. The physician's real question is how to manage this patient with asymptomatic hyperuricemia, and the answer given above is not appropriate for this specific problem. A more useful response would be the following:

Hydrochlorothiazide (in Esimil®) is well documented to produce asymptomatic or symptomatic hyperuricemia when given in low doses.[1,2] The incidence of hyperuricemia in hypertensive patients receiving thiazides is reported to be 65-70 percent, as compared to an incidence of 25-30 percent in untreated primary hypertensive patients with normal renal function.[3,4] It is probable that this patient is presenting with hyperuricemia secondary to thiazide administration. Thiazide-induced increases in serum uric acid can occur within a few days of therapy and are usually asymptomatic. Serum uric acid levels usually return to normal soon after the thiazides are discontinued. However, whether the hyperuricemia in this patient is thiazide-induced or due to other reasons, allopurinol should effectively lower serum uric acid levels. Nicotero[5] reported that allopurinol 300 mg daily effectively prevented the hyperuricemia produced by chlorothiazide 1 g daily, with serum uric acid levels maintained below pre-thiazide levels. Allopurinol did not interfere with the hypotensive effects of chlorothiazide.

The question here is really whether or not to treat asymptomatic hyperuricemia secondary to thiazide administration or other causes. Unfortunately, there are no firm guidelines as to who should be treated, since there are no definitive studies to indicate the fate of untreated patients with asymptomatic hyperuricemia. Patients should not be exposed to the unnecessary risks of adverse drug reactions of hyperuricemic agents when a high percentage will never experience an acute attack of gout. However, if serum uric acid levels are consistently elevated between 9–10 mg%, drug therapy is indicated regardless of the cause. The Framingham Study[6] showed that in populations with serum uric acid levels greater than 9 mg%, approximately 83 percent are likely to develop gouty arthritis. Therapy is aimed at preventing both tophaceous joint deposits as well as uric acid renal deposits.

Conclusion. The possibility of thiazide-induced hyperuricemia should be considered in this patient. If the patient is to continue Esimil®, she should be treated with Zyloprim®, since serum uric acid levels exceed 9 mg%. There is no evidence that this combination will result in decreased hypotensive effects. Discontinuing the Esimil® (and thus the thiazide) should result in the lowering of uric acid levels in a short period if the hyperuricemia is drug-induced. There are no other clinically significant interactions in the patient's regimen.

References

1. Healey, L.A. et al.: Uric Acid Retention Due to Hydrochlorothiazide, *N.Engl.J.Med.* 261:1358, 1959
2. Aronoff, A. and Barkum, H.: Hyperuricemia and Acute Gouty Arthritis Precipitated by Thiazide Derivatives, *Can.Med.Assoc.J.* 84:1181, 1961
3. Cannon, P.J. et al.: Hyperuricemia in Primary and Renal Hypertension, *N.Engl.J.Med.* 275:457–464, 1966
4. Breckenridge, A.: Hypertension and Hyperuricemia, *Lancet* 1:15–18, 1966
5. Nicotero, J.A. et al.: Prevention of Hyperuricemia by Allopurinol in Hypertensive Patients Treated with Chlorothiazide, *N.Engl.J.Med.* 282:133–135, 1970
6. Hall, A.P. et al.: Epidemiology of Gout and Hyperuricemia, *Am.J.Med.* 42:27–37, 1967

It can be seen that appropriate background information can completely modify the nature of the response that the pharmacist should provide. Therefore, formulation and communication of the response must be organized to meet the needs of the caller, so that the answer given will be relevant and useful. This requires an understanding of *why* the question is being asked.

Formulating the Response

There are no standardized guidelines for formulating a response. Almost every drug information pharmacist develops individualized techniques for written responses. However, the student new to providing drug information should follow some technique when first approaching questions; the development of specialized or individual techniques can be promulgated from this basic approach. The following guidelines may be useful when formulating a response for either a verbal or written reply.

1. Evaluate and list all references searched in an attempt to find the information.

2. Write down statements from the references which are pertinent to the answer.
Reference this information appropriately.

3. Using this information, prepare a summary to answer the question.
This summary should be concise and pertinent to the request and its circumstances.

4. It is sometimes necessary to include detailed or peripheral information to explain part of the answer.
Indepth or very detailed information is not necessary unless indicated, however. The quality of a response depends upon how well the applicable information is summarized into usable form, not on how long the answer is.

5. Be prepared to respond to other questions from the caller when presenting the answer.
For example, if the caller wants to know the drug of choice for a urinary tract infection, be prepared to suggest alternative drugs with appropriate doses.

6. Present a verbal reply and/or prepare a formal written response.

Most drug information centers supply both verbal and written responses. The rule is usually that a verbal response is supplied first (in the time specified) and this is then followed by a written answer. Written responses are generally supplied when: (1) the request required a great deal of research and preparation; (2) the answer is of sufficient value to keep for future reference; or (3) a written reply is requested by the inquirer.

Although the format of the answer may differ for certain types of questions, the following format represents a good basis for an adequately structured response:

Request and Background Information
This should be a brief statement of the problem and its circumstances.

Response
1. *Introduction or background.* In some cases a brief introductory opening is necessary for clarification of the terminology, issues at hand, etc.
2. *Finding.* Summarize what the literature says about the problem. Any inadequacies and deficiencies of the studies or references cited should also be noted. Be concise, unbiased and above all accurate.
3. *Tables, graphs, charts.* Include, where appropriate, any tables, graphs and charts (original or otherwise) that will assist and clarify the literature findings.

Conclusion
Briefly summarize what has been found with appropriate conclusions. This portion of the response should answer the request; everything written in the finding should merely substantiate the answer or conclusion. In addition, this portion of the response should include any recommendation, alteration, or adjustments in the management of the requestor's problems.

References
All significant and important statements in the main body of the report should be footnoted. To re-emphasize, any unreferenced statement of fact is for all practical purposes useless. Reference citings should follow a standard format (see Chapter 1), the use of which will facilitate an organized and "pharmaceutically elegant" written drug information report. In addition, the correct rules of grammar, syntax, punctuation, and spelling must always be observed (Strunk, 1972). See Chapter 8 for examples of style and format for written answers. *The Medical Letter on Drug & Therapeutics* also represents an excellent role-model for well-written, concise texts.

Communicating the Response

Communication of the response is accomplished verbally in all cases and supplemented by written material in certain instances. Not all questions will require the use of the guidelines and format for a written response as discussed previously. Although many questions will require research and thus necessitate calling the inquirer back, some questions may be answered while the inquirer is still on the telephone. Examples of questions of this nature include:

1. Intravenous incompatibility;
2. Simple dosing recommendations or calculations;
3. Drug identification or availability;
4. Foreign or investigational drug identification;
5. Poisonings; and
6. Questions previously answered that are readily available.

The following guidelines may assist the student or practitioner when communicating a verbal response.

1. If a specific answer cannot be found, an answer should not be guessed at or bluffed.

2. The statement "There have been no reports in the literature" cannot be made until all available reference sources have been adequately searched.

3. Information should be prepared in a logical sequence using the guidelines listed above before calling the inquirer.

It is unprofessional to fumble through references in an attempt to find an answer while a caller is waiting on the telephone.

4. Statements such as "I think," or "I don't think" are not appropriate when presenting an answer.

The confidence displayed when giving a response is an important communication skill in providing drug information. The confidence the caller has in the services a pharmacist provides depends on the accuracy, as well as the confidence displayed when an answer is presented. For example, it is preferable to say "There are no reports in the literature of renal damage due to drug X," than "I don't think drug X can cause renal damage."

5. The inquirer should be contacted within the time specified, even though the question may not have been answered.

It is appropriate to call back even if it is just to indicate that additional time is required to research an answer. Dependability is essential to developing credibility.

6. Abstracts (de Haen system, FDA abstracts) alone should never be used when communicating a response.

An attempt should always be made to obtain the original article, since abstracts often contain statements out of context which may not be descriptive of the true contents or meaning of the study.

7. The caller should be asked if the information provided was what he needed or required.

Occasionally an answer provided by the pharmacist is not what was specifically required by the caller. This frequently occurs when insufficient background information has been obtained by the pharmacist.

8. The caller should be asked if additional information is required on the subject, as well as if a written response is desired.

9. If a question is answered relatively quickly because of the caller's urgency, present an initial answer and state that if additional information or data are found that would modify the initial answer, a return call will be made.

10. Keep calling the inquirer back until both you and he are satisfied with the answer.

This is important and will be a deciding factor in signifying the success of a drug information specialist.

Follow-up

Once the answer has been communicated it is important to follow-up whenever possible, especially for patient-specific questions. Follow-up is recommended for several reasons.

1. To determine if the right question was in fact asked and if the right answer was given.

This is usually determined when the response is given, but may not be evident in some cases until follow-up is performed.

2. To determine if the answer or recommendation was accepted and if there was any impact on patient care.

This is essential in order to determine the value of providing drug information services, as well as to provide positive or negative feedback on the outcome of the answer.

3. To determine if further assistance can be given.

This is especially important in patient-related situations. An answer given in one instance may be satisfactory, whereas half an hour later a totally different situation may have developed. For example, a call regarding an alcoholic patient with severe cirrhosis who is in a prehepatic coma state is received. The question concerns the effectiveness of lactulose to prevent further increases in serum ammonia levels. After an answer is presented, the patient goes into frank hepatic coma. At this point the pharmacist should be available to present further recommendations, such as the use of levo-dopa for hepatic coma.

The essence of this chapter is that the pharmacist should provide answers that meet the *specific needs* of the caller and not just factual data about drugs or drug therapy. This requires: an insight into the caller's circumstances at the time of the request; determination of "what the caller *really* wants to know;" followed by the provision of concise, usable, information.

Background Reading

1. Hirschman, J.L. and Maudlin, R.K.: Drug Information Analysis Service— The DIAS Rounds, *Drug Intell.Clin.Pharm.* 4:10–12, 1970
2. Hirschman, J.L. and Maudlin, R.K.: The DIAS Rounds, *Drug Intell. Clin. Pharm.* 4:149–152, 1970
3. Strunk, W. and White, E.B.: *Elements of Style*, 2nd Ed., Macmillan Co., New York, N.Y., 1972
4. Beatty, W.K.: Searching the Literature Comes Before Writing the Literature, *Ann.Intern.Med.* 79:917–924, 1973
5. *The Medical Letter on Drugs and Therapeutics*, The Medical Letter, Inc., 56 Harrison Street, New Rochelle, N.Y.

Self Evaluation Questions and Learning Examples on How to Formulate and Communicate a Response

6.1 Which skills will be useful in formulating a response to a drug information request?
6.2 Which parameters are essential to the format of a written response?
6.3 Identify ten guidelines that will assist in the provision of better verbal responses to drug information questions.
6.4 Identify three points that indicate the rationale for providing drug information request follow-up response calls.
6.5 *Learning Examples.* Identify the classification type and missing background and history information, then prepare a written response utilizing the recommended format for the following case examples. The key to these examples is in the "Case Histories" located in Chapter 8.

a. Is clindamycin considered the drug of choice for suspected *Clostridia* infections?
b. How prevalent is ampicillin-resistant *Haemophilus Influenzae* meningitis? Should chloramphenicol be considered the drug of choice for ampicillin-resistant *Haemophilus Influenzae* meningitis? What other antibiotics have been used?
c. What are the characteristics of phenothiazine-induced leukopenia?
d. Can nitrofurantoin cause leukocytosis and fever?
e. Can quinidine produce fever and rashes?
f. Will one gram daily doses of Keflex® achieve adequate urinary concentrations in the presence of uremia?
g. What is the maximum daily dose of chloramphenicol for *H. Influenzae* meningitis?
h. What is Propirina®?
i. Can Gelusil® increase the absorption of anticonvulsants and result in increased anticonvulsant serum levels?
j. In a patient presenting with digitalis toxicity, how long must you wait before giving another dose? What should the maintenance dose be?
k. Are blood levels obtained from oral chloramphenicol palmitate lower than levels obtained with IV chloramphenicol? If so, what dose of the oral preparation must be given to produce equivalent blood levels?
l. What is in Tri-Aqua® and is it toxic?
m. What symptoms can be expected from chewing leaves of the plant Dumb Cane?

7

Situations and Problems in Providing Drug Information

Behavioral Objectives for Chapter Seven Situations and Problems in Providing Drug Information

OBJECTIVE	CRITERIA FOR MEETING OBJECTIVE	SELF EVALUATION QUESTION NUMBER
The student should be able to:	The student should be able to discuss:	
7.1 Demonstrate an awareness of the practical approaches to specific situations and problems in providing drug information	7.1.1 Specific problem situations relating to searching the literature 7.1.11 Use of textbooks 7.1.12 Use of abstracts 7.1.13 Use of earlier literature 7.1.14 Use of the most current literature 7.1.15 No data found in the literature 7.1.16 The complete search	7.1 7.2 7.4 7.6
	7.1.2 Utilizing Non-literature information sources 7.1.21 Use of specialists and agencies 7.1.22 Use of the drug manufacturers	7.3 7.6
	7.1.3 Formulating a response 7.1.31 Written response 7.1.32 Use of tables and graphs 7.1.33 Conflicting reports in the literature 7.1.34 Disease state background knowledge	7.4 7.6

Behavioral Objectives for Chapter Seven Situations and Problems in Providing Drug Information (*continued*)

OBJECTIVE	CRITERIA FOR MEETING OBJECTIVE	SELF EVALUATION QUESTION NUMBER

7.1 Demonstrate an awareness of the practical approaches to specific situations and problems in providing drug information (*continued*)	7.1.4 Specific Problems
	    7.1.41 Problems with synonyms, indexing and medical terminology
	    7.1.42 The News Media
	    7.1.43 Teratogenicity
	    7.1.43 Investigational Drugs
		7.5
		7.6

General Discussion

Previous chapter discussions have provided the novice drug information student or practitioner with guidelines to learning and applying a systematic approach to the answering of drug information requests. This chapter will acquaint the student with specific situations and problems commonly encountered during the provision of drug information services. It includes methods of utilizing different information sources, additional practical guidelines for the formulation of responses, and approaches to specific types of questions not previously discussed. The application of the systematic approach to these situations and examples will familiarize the student with some of the techniques and methodologies used in a drug information service. The illustrative case histories and examples described in this chapter also contain the dates the questions were received and worked up.

Problem Situations in Searching the Literature

Use of Textbooks

Many questions can be answered over the telephone with the use of reference texts and thus the need to search or use the primary literature is bypassed. Questions of this type include: (1) drug identification; (2) drug availability; (3) pharmaceutical compatibility; (4) poisoning; and (5) drug dosing.

Textbooks, with their large factual data base, can also be useful in answering specific patient-related problems and questions. However, it is important to note that many questions dealing with specific patients require responses based on current primary literature. The following example illustrates a specific patient request answered with the use of textbooks. In this example, the information cited in the texts was referenced to journals in a foreign language, thus making the use of the reference text mandatory, in lieu of the original articles.

Request. (1/20/75) A 23-year-old male received smallpox, diphtheria, cholera, tetanus and typhoid vaccines on 1/15/75 in preparation for travelling abroad. He developed lower back pains, muscle aches, fever, headache and hematuria 24–48 hours later. Urinalysis at this time revealed 4+ albumin, 100 RBC's/hpf, coffee-colored urine. Past Hx: Glomerulonephritis at age 2; received Diphtheria-Tetanus Toxoid 4 years ago. Is this an allergic response to the vaccines? What should be done?

Response. The symptoms of fever, headache, myalgia, and general malaise can be caused by diphtheria toxoid, typhoid vaccine, cholera vaccine, or a combination of all 3 of the above.[1,2] The patient's urinary symptoms, however, could only be caused by typhoid vaccine or diphtheria toxoid. Smallpox vaccine has been reported to elicit a nephrotic syndrome, but this is rare and symptoms would not appear until 10–12 days after injection.[1] The occurrence of nephritis or a nephrotic syndrome due to vaccination with TABDT (typhoid fever, paratyphoid fever A & B, diphtheria, tetanus) vaccine was observed in 33 cases in a military hospital between 1952 and 1958. All showed an allergic reaction to some component of the combined vaccine.[2]

The patient's urinalysis (hematuria, 4+ albumin) as well as his lumbar pain and general malaise suggest a glomerulonephritis. It is possible that the typhoid or diphtheria vaccines could have reactivated this patient's childhood glomerulonephritis. There is no specific treatment for this condition; only symptomatic prevention of overhydration and hypertension can be monitored. Adrenocorticosteroids and corticotropin are of no value and may be contraindicated because they increase protein catabolism, sodium retention and hypertension.[3]

A final possibility is that the patient may be exhibiting Shwartzman's Syndrome, which is characterized by cortical necrosis of the kidneys triggered by intravascular coagulation of blood.[4] One case of Shwartzman's Syndrome has been reported after revaccination of a 22-year-old man with TABDT vaccine.[5] This possibility should be considered, although it is very rare.

The patient should not be exposed again to typhoid or diphtheria vaccines, since severe complications could arise.

References

1. Meyler, L. (Ed.): *Side Effects of Drugs, Vol. VII.* Excerpta Medica Foundation, New York, 1972, pp. 445–449
2. Meyler, L. (Ed.): *Side Effects of Drugs, Vol. IV.* Excerpta Medica Foundation, New York, p. 316
3. Krupp, M.A. et al. (Eds.): *Current Diagnosis and Treatment,* Lange Medical Publications, Los Altos California, 1973, pp. 513–515
4. Perry, T.M. and Miller, F.N. (Eds.): *Pathology,* 2nd edition. Little, Brown and Company, Boston, 1961, p. 88
5. Meyler, L. (Ed.): *Side Effects of Drugs, Vol. V.* Williams and Wilkins Company, Maryland, 1966, p. 377

Use of Abstracts

Generally, abstracts such as *de Haen, Clin Alert* or *International Pharmaceutical Abstracts (IPA)* should never be used alone to answer drug information requests, particularly for patient-related questions. The reason for this is that abstracts may contain out of context statements and may not always provide enough information to indicate the true content of the original article.

However, if an article is published in a foreign language and a translation is not readily available, an abstract, if used with appropriate caution, may be useful. Similarly, if an abstract from either a domestic or foreign journal is the only data found in the literature on the subject, then cautious use of the abstract would be permissible. In all other situations, the original article should be retrieved and evaluated. A very useful abstracting service for drug information centers is *de Haen Drugs in Use*, which outlines the study's data and results and allows the reader to obtain a more detailed overview of the article's contents. Narrative abstracts are less useful (e.g., *IPA, Excerpta Medica Abstracts*) in this regard.

An example of a situation where abstracts are useful in a patient-related question follows.

Request. (3/8/74) A 41-year-old female has developed pneumonia secondary to *Pseudomonas aeruginosa*. She has been receiving gentamicin 80 mg IM qid for 9 days and is defervescing. She now has evidence of pancytopenia, as seen by a recent WBC of 2000, anemia and thrombocytopenia; results of a bone marrow biopsy are not completed. Can gentamicin cause pancytopenia? Should we leave the patient on the drug?

Response. Bone marrow depression and pancytopenia are certainly not well-documented adverse effects of gentamicin. Clinical investigations have not associated gentamicin with hematopoietic toxicity and most authoritative references indicate that no changes in hematological functions have been cited from the use of the drug.[1,2] However, other sources indicate that gentamicin has been reported on very rare occasions to cause a reversible depression of granulocytes and a decreased hematocrit. Also reported rarely are thrombocytopenia, anemia and increased or decreased reticulocyte count, all of which are apparently reversible.[3-5] We have not, however, been able to document all of these effects in clinical reports.

A thorough search of the literature revealed only two reports of blood dyscrasias associated with gentamicin.[6,7] These cases describe the occurrence of acute agranulocytosis, but a definite cause-effect relationship and other specific information about the patients involved could not be established, as both studies are in a foreign language. However, other aminoglycosides (kanamycin and streptomycin) have been associated with bone marrow suppression and in this context gentamicin could be considered to have the propensity to cause marrow suppression and associated granulocytopenia with or without pancytopenia, however rare the effect may be.

The renal disease in this patient may itself be a cause of the marrow suppression, but gentamicin should be considered until proven otherwise, even though the evidence is relatively scarce. If significant renal impairment exists, gentamicin blood levels at this dose are probably in the toxic range and this may have been a contributing factor. At this point gentamicin should probably be discontinued, in order to rule out or confirm its contribution to the apparently developing pancytopenia, as its hematological effects should be reversible. Although penicillins are not free of toxic effect on the bone marrow, including agranulocytosis and pancytopenia, the substitution of carbenicillin for gentamicin would probably be a prudent choice if *Pseudomonas* is definitely the causative organism. Dosage of carbenicillin should be reduced, based on the severity of the renal impairment, to avoid accumulation and toxicity.

References

1. Kucers, A.: *The Use of Antibiotics.* William Heinemann, Ltd., London, 1972, p. 146

2. Cox, C.E.: Gentamicin, *Med. Clin. North Am.* 54:1305–1314, 1970

3. Arcieri, G.M. et al.: Clinical Research Experience with Gentamicin—Incidence of Adverse Reactions, *Med. J. Aust.*, 1 (Suppl): 30–34, 1974

4. AMA Council on Drugs: *AMA Drug Evaluations*, 2nd Ed., Publishing Sciences Grp., Acton, Mass., 1973, p. 570

5. *American Hospital Formulary Service*, Am. Soc. Hosp. Pharm., Washington, 8:12.28 (Gentamicin)

6. Walbaum, R. et al.: A Case of Acute Agranulocytosis, *Lille. Medicale* 16:1074–1075, 1971 (French)

7. Ruvidik, R.: Drug-Induced Acute Agranulocytosis, *Srpski. Arkh. Tselok. Lek.* 100:101–108, 1972 (Yugoslavian)

Use of the Earlier Literature

As a general rule, a search of the literature over the past ten to twelve years is sufficient to provide an adequate response to many questions. Most pharmacists or drug information centers have neither the time nor the reference capability to search past this point on a routine basis. However, some drug information questions cannot be answered due to the lack of any "recent" literature. Examples of questions of this nature include: "Can carbon monoxide exposure cause symptoms of Parkinsonism?" or "How clinically significant is the tetracycline-milk interaction? Are there any studies documenting significantly decreased tetracycline serum levels in patients as a result of the interaction?" Most of the literature written on these subjects was published in the 1950's and earlier. Usually, appropriate textbooks can assist in locating many of the original reference citations and minimize the need to search the early literature. Unfortunately however, not all references for these kinds of questions can be obtained from textbooks and as a result the pharmacist will occasionally be required to search the earlier literature.

If a drug or therapeutic procedure has not been mentioned in the literature within the last ten to fifteen years, there is the possibility that it has been proved ineffective, or that its use has waned through lack of interest or documented efficacy. The following question is an example of this.

Request. (5/1/74) We have heard of the histamine test to detect certain types of nerve damage, specifically sympathetic nervous system damage. How is this test administered and how do you evaluate the response?

Response. The cutaneous reaction to histamine is a triple response which consists of an initial red reaction (primary flare), and the formation of a localized wheal, followed by the appearance of an extended area of arterial dilatation—the flare.[1,2] The histamine test is based on the presumption that the flare phenomenon is attributed to a neurogenic mechanism mediated by the peripheral nerve supply. Specifically, this involves antidromic transmission (axon reflex) along sensory fibers[1,3] and perhaps the involvement of a suprasegmental reflex arc, the afferent arm of which reaches as high as the diencephalon.[2] Neither the preganglionic sympathetic fibers nor the final common pathway are essential to the spreading flare, and it is suggested that both afferent and efferent impulses in this reflex travel via sensory nerves and dorsal nerve routes.[3] Lack of the spreading flare reaction to intradermal histamine would indicate damage to peripheral nerves. The test was described by Loeser[1] in 1938. Since the 1:1000 histamine HCl suggested by Loeser is no longer available, histamine PO_4 1:10,000 may be used. The dose recommended is 0.1 ml of a 1:10,000 solution injected intradermally. Several injections may be given from 1–3 inches apart across the area to be tested. Reactions are graded on a scale of 0–4, according to the amount and intensity of the flare: A wheal with no flare is 0. A wheal surrounded by an intense flare (at 30 min) is a 4+. The wheal usually forms is 20 seconds to 1 minute. The flare, if it forms, should reach its height in 3–5 minutes and begin to fade in 7–10 minutes. Loeser described several uses of the histamine test for appraisal of peripheral nerve function.

It should be mentioned that the histamine test for nerve function is not approved by the FDA nor by the Eli Lilly Company. Communication with Eli Lilly revealed that their research in this area is extremely limited and that no studies are currently on file discussing the technique. Based upon limited clinical use, as well as inadequate documentation of its efficacy in the literature, the histamine test is at present considered to be of dubious value.

References

1. Loeser, L.H.: The Cutaneous Histamine Reaction as a Test of Peripheral Nerve Function, *J. Am. Med. Assoc.*: June 25, 1938

2. Cooper, I.S.: A Neurologic Evaluation of the Cutaneous Histamine Reaction, *J. Clin. Invest.* 29:465–469, 1970

3. Smith, Alfred and Dancis, J.: Response to Intradermal Histamine in Familial Dysautonomia—A Diagnostic Test, *J. Pediatr.* 63:889–894, 1963

There are certain questions for which recent reports have described the inadequacy of a drug based on the earlier literature, thus searching out the earlier reports may not be necessary in some cases. Most of these questions will involve the work of the federal agencies which brought about the withdrawal of the drug from the market. The following is such an example.

Request. (2/29/76) How effective is Neutrapen® (penicillinase) in the treatment of allergic reactions to penicillin, specifically anaphylaxis?

Response. The administration of penicillinase reportedly results in the "rapid" destruction of circulating penicillin. However, penicillinase is no longer on the market due to its purported lack of efficacy.[1,2] Although the drug may lower penicillin G serum levels, there is no evidence that this in itself is useful for the treatment of allergic reactions to penicillin. There are no clinical studies evaluating the effectiveness of penicillinase since 1962, and most of the clinical work involving the drug was performed prior to this period. To our knowledge, there are very few studies available regarding the efficacy of penicillinase. The ones available apparently do not represent adequate and well-controlled trials. The effects of penicillinase are seen several hours after injection and they are of no benefit to the patient suffering an anaphylactic reaction to penicillin.

In addition, penicillinase is not without risk itself, because of its own sensitizing potential. Anaphylactic reactions following the administration of penicillinase have been reported; penicillinase may itself act as a protein antigen or there may be foreign protein in the commercial product. For these reasons we cannot recommend the use of penicillinase for any type of penicillin reaction.

References
1. Randolph, W.: Penicillinase Injection, *Federal Register* 38:34354, 1973
2. Krout, J.: Penicillinase Injection, *Federal Register* 40:44599, 1975

Use of the Most Current Literature

The lag period for most secondary literature sources can vary from as short as three months to as long as a year or more, depending on the source used (see table in Chapter Four). This presents a problem for the pharmacist, who must conduct a complete literature search that includes all recent studies. Obtaining recent studies is most significant when dealing with patient-specific consultations, and one measure of the value of the drug information service will be based upon the provision of up-to-date, as well as accurate, information. This problem is overcome by the use of the following three secondary reference sources; most drug information centers have access to at least one of these sources in order to keep abreast of current literature.

InPharma

InPharma is a weekly publication presenting abstracts from 1700 journals throughout the world. Each week, abstracts are presented covering all major areas of drugs, i.e., adverse reactions, drug therapy, pharmacology, research and development etc. In addition, bibliographies on various subjects or specific drugs from the recent literature are also published. A quarterly index allows entry into the system. The lag period for *InPharma* is two weeks to three months.

MEDLINE and TOXLINE

MEDLINE is Medlars on line and provides computer access to the entire *Index Medicus* data base (2500 journals), *Index to Drug Literature* and *International Nursing Index* covering the previous three years (see Chapter Four). The inherent lag period for MEDLINE may be from one to three months, which is significantly shorter than the printed index's lag period of up to a year or longer. MEDLINE provides a computerized printout on a specific topic prior to the printing of this information in the monthly issue of *Index Medicus*. TOXLINE covers all reports on adverse effects and toxicity in *Index Medicus*, plus other pertinent abstracting services in the area of toxicity and adverse effects (*Chemical-Biological Activities, Health Effects of Environmental Pollutants, International Pharmaceutical Abstracts, Pesticide Abstracts* and *Hayes File on Pesticides*). TOXLINE is very useful for locating recent information on adverse drug reactions. There is usually a fee (which varies from state to state) for utilizing MEDLINE or TOXLINE.

Current Contents—Clinical Practice

This reference lists the table of contents for over 725 medical and related journals on a weekly basis. Each issue's subject index allows the pharmacist to locate recent drug or disease articles. Access to the index of all issues of *Current Contents* for a period of three to six months enables one to search the literature over this period of time. This process is often time consuming, but can be of considerable assistance in overcoming the lag period inherent to other secondary sources.

The following example is a question for which *Current Contents—Clinical Practice* was utilized to formulate the response. Note the amount of time between the date of the request and reference number one by Dalessio in the *Journal of the American Medical Association*. This reference may have been overlooked without the assistance of this secondary source.

Request. (11/29/73) We have a 49-year-old male with trigeminal neuralgia who has been fairly well controlled on Tegretol® 1000 mg/day (5 tabs) for three years. However, he has developed chronic, severe diarrhea in the past three weeks which has become incapacitating.

1. Are there any new developments in the drug therapy of trigeminal neuralgia?

2. Can Tegretol® cause a severe diarrhea late in the course of therapy?

Response. 1. The most recent therapy proposed for trigeminal neuralgia is that of Dalessio.[1] He used chlorphenesin carbamate (Maolate®) in 4 patients with trigeminal neuralgia in doses of 1600 mg daily

(400 mg am, 400 mg at noon, 800 mg hs). This resulted in prompt reduction in the sensitivity of facial trigger zones, followed in 1–2 days by loss of the typical lancinating pain of trigeminal neuralgia. He also reported that 2 patients only partially responding to diphenylhydantoin or carbamazepine, or both, improved somewhat with the addition of chlorphenesin. However, the duration of treatment, side effects and follow-up were not provided, thus limiting the clinical significance of the report. More controlled studies are needed.

Chlorphenesin is an old drug and one not without side effects. Drowsiness, dizziness, nausea, epigastric distress, constipation, headache and euphoria have been reported.[2] Hepatotoxicity has been reported in animals, but changes in liver function in humans have not been attributed to the drug. However, liver function tests should be monitored during prolonged therapy. Paradoxical reactions of nervousness, insomnia and hyperexcitability have also been reported.

2. Long-term controlled studies to evaluate the side effects of chronic usage of carbamazepine (Tegretol®) have not been reported. Although diarrhea is listed as a common side effect of the drug, we failed to substantiate this in the literature. Of 305 patients receiving the drug over various periods of time, only 7 developed diarrhea.[4–8] However, in 2 of these cases, drug discontinuation was necessary.[4,6] Arieff and Wetzel[7] reported mild diarrhea after several months of therapy in one patient who had taken between 100–800 mg daily. Since no other etiology was apparent, the patient continued taking Tegretol® despite the persistent diarrhea. Of all studies reviewed, this was the only one that specifically mentioned at what point in therapy the diarrhea occurred, and this was vague at best. It is our contention that diarrhea occurs more frequently with Tegretol® than is reported in the literature. When it does occur, it may be severe enough and persistent enough to warrant discontinuation of therapy.

References

1. Dalessio, D.J.: Chlorphenesin for Trigeminal Neuralgia, *J. Am. Med. Assoc.*, 225:1659 (Sept. 24) 1973

2. Meyler, L. and Herxheimer, A.: *Side Effects of Drugs, Vol. 7*, Excerpta Medica, Amsterdam, 1972, p. 68

3. *American Hospital Formulary Service*, Am. Soc. Hosp. Pharm., Washington, 12:20 (Chlorphenesin)

4. Graham, J.G. and Zilkha, K.J.: Treatment of Trigeminal Neuralgia with Carbamazepine: A Follow-Up Study, *Br. Med. J.* 1:210–211, 1966

5. Lloyd-Smith, D.L. and Sachdev, K.K.: A Long-Term Low-Dosage Study of Carbamazepine in Trigeminal Neuralgia, *Headache* 9:64–72, 1969

6. Heathfield, K. and Colin-Jones, D.G.: Treatment of Trigeminal Neuralgia with Tegretol®, *Br. Med. J.* 1:481, 1966

7. Arieff, A.J. and Wetzel, N.: Tegretol® in the Treatment of Neuralgias, *Dis. Nerv. Syst.* 28:820–823, 1967

8. Dalessio, D.J.: Medical Treatment of Tic Douloureux, *J. Chronic Dis.* 19:1043–1048, 1966

Follow-up. The Tegretol® was discontinued with a corresponding abatement of the diarrhea. At the same time, Maolate® 1600 mg daily was instituted. As of January 1974, the patient had responded well to the Maolate® with a great reduction of the amount of pain. Thus far he has not complained of any side effects of the drug.

When Data Cannot be Found in the Literature

In some situations a complete literature search reveals no specific information relevant to answering a drug question. Stating "there have been no reports in the literature" is one response approach; however, in some cases the pharmacist may want to provide some information with appropriate qualification, whether or not substantiating reports were found. For example, if a search of the literature concerning a drug and an adverse reaction is conclusive, it is probably safe to rule out the drug as having caused the adverse reaction on the basis that it has not been documented or reported. However, this does not mean the agent is not responsible, but that it is unlikely that it is. Other situations occur where no precise answer exists in the literature and the pharmacist must use his experience and knowledge to analyse and interpret the applicable information in order to postulate or theorize a reasonable explanation. For example, if the caller desires to know how drug X is metabolized and excreted and this data is unavailable, the pharmacist may be able to extrapolate pharmacokinetic parameters from other similar therapeutic agents and thus make a reasonable "guess." It is important to note that extrapolation is frequently an inaccurate method, but in situations pertaining to closely related drugs in the same species, i.e., man, it is justified.

Occasionally, situations arise which could lead one to believe there is no literature available, when in fact the desired data were not found because of an erroneous search. A good example of this is the improper use of indexing terms and synonyms; this error is mentioned in a later discussion in this chapter. Another example is the misspelling of terms and names. Although this type of error appears self-evident, experience has shown that questions are sometimes not answered (or no data are found to answer the questions) because the drug or disease state was misspelled, either by the inquirer or the person receiving the call, thus leading to an unproductive search. This occurs mainly with foreign or investigational drugs and uncommon disease states. A good medical dictionary (Stedman's) and a text such as *Pharmacological and Chemical Synonyms* (Marler) are valuable aids in preventing these types of mix up.

Questions may also involve the use of drugs or therapeutic procedures that have been mentioned at recent medical symposia or conferences, for which there is no published data in the literature. If, however, it is ascertained from the caller where the meeting was held and who presented the material, this will facilitate a response based on data obtained by contacting the individual who made the presentation at that meeting. In addition, contacting the manufacturer of the drug in question can be a useful source of relevant unpublished data.

The Complete Search

Many pharmacists have a tendency to answer requests using the "off the top of the head" approach, i.e., answering questions without appropriate research or documentation. It is important to remember that there is always the possibility that there is information that the pharmacist is not aware of. Therefore, unless the pharmacist knows from previous research and experience with the drugs in question, he is obligated to do a literature search. However, it is not always practical or possible for the pharmacist to conduct a thorough or complete search for every question. Therefore, certain guidelines and judgments from previous experience can assist in determining what constitutes an appropriate search.

Although a complete literature search implies that every possible information source has been covered, practice dictates that a "complete" search depends on the type of question. For example, a complete search of the literature for a drug identification question often covers different sources to one for an adverse drug reaction or therapeutic question. In addition, from a logistical viewpoint, a complete search depends on what access to the drug literature a pharmacist has.

Most questions do not require a complete or thorough literature search, since an adequate search of specific sources, depending on the type of question, will provide adequate information. The following secondary literature source listing for specific types of questions represents reasonable guidelines for a "complete" literature search. Assuming that the appropriate reference texts have been consulted (see Chapter Four), an unproductive search through these sources would indicate the likelihood of there being no reports in the literature.

Drug Therapy or Efficacy, Pharmacokinetic and Dosing Questions

de Haen Drugs in Use
Iowa Drug Information System
Index Medicus (to 1960)
International Pharmaceutical Abstracts
Excerpta Medica Specialty Abstracts
Recent literature. Current Contents—Clinical Practice, InPharma, MEDLINE computer search

Drug Identification or Availability Questions
  de Haen Drugs in Research (and Drugs in Use)
  Iowa Drug Information System
  Chemical Abstracts
  Excerpta Medica Drug Literature Index
  Unlisted Drugs
  Pharm-Index
  Foreign compendia for specific country

Adverse Drug Reactions/Drug Interactions Questions
  de Haen Drugs in Use
  Iowa Drug Information System
  Clin-Alert
  FDA Clinical Experience Abstracts
  Adverse Reaction Titles
  Index Medicus
  Toxicity Bibliography
  Recent literature: Current Contents—Clinical Practice, InPharma
    TOXLINE computer search

For most poisoning cases a complete search of the literature is not indicated, since the information response required must be immediate (see Chapter Four for Poisoning References). However, for cases of chronic poisonings (e.g., peripheral neuropathy from prolonged exposure to 2,4-D), then a complete search may be conducted and the same sources that are listed for adverse drug reaction questions must be consulted. There are some instances of acute poisonings where, *after* providing the initial toxicity and treatment data, the literature can be consulted to find cases correlating to the one in question. Good sources for this include: de Haen Drugs in Use, FDA Clinical Experience Abstracts, Clin-Alert and Toxicity Bibliography.

The following is an example of a response given when no information was found following a "complete" search:

Request. (11/29/73) We have two patients on phenformin who have recently presented with asymptomatic hyperuricemia (uric acid 8–10 mg percent). Both are receiving doses of 50 mg bid. Can DBI-TD® be the cause of increased uric acid levels?

Response. A thorough search of the literature revealed no reports of hyperuricemia from phenformin. Except for two isolated cases of azotemia,[1] phenformin apparently lacks nephrotoxic potential. No clinical symptoms or histological findings of renal damage have been reported in man, and urate retention cannot be attributed to phenformin nephrotoxicity.

Phenformin is most likely not the cause of the observed hyperuricemias; gout has been associated with diabetes mellitus and this is more likely the case in these patients.

References

1. Menon, I.S. and Dewar, H.A.: Increased Blood-Urea During Phenformin Therapy, *Lancet* 2:263, 1970

Utilizing Other Information Sources

Use of Specialists and Agencies

On occasion it is useful to utilize specialists. Specialists may be helpful: (1) to provide any recent drug therapy information in specific patient-related questions that may not be published in the literature; and (2) to, on occasion, verify documented literature findings. For example, a question such as "Has indigo carmine ever been used intrathecally to detect cerebral spinal fluid leaks?" may require consultation with a neurologist who may have used this procedure in his practice or is familiar with its use in other institutions. On other occasions, obtaining a consultation from an appropriate specialist with regard to a specific problem, e.g., an adverse drug reaction, is helpful when very little literature is available on the subject.

Certain national agencies, e.g., the Food and Drug Administration (FDA), the Center for Disease Control in Atlanta and the Public Health Service, are also helpful in providing information on the use of investigational drugs, vaccines and drug therapy for less well known diseases.

The pharmacist should utilize these resources, since information obtained from such specialists and agencies can help provide a more useful, up-to-date response.

Use of The Drug Manufacturer

Most major drug manufacturers maintain extensive data files on their products, as well as unpublished anecdotal and clinical reports from physicians and project investigators regarding the use of their drugs in patients. In addition, many drug manufacturers also have a clinical pharmacologist in charge of a particular area, e.g., infectious disease, who may be another useful information source on a drug product. The pharmacist may find the manufacturer helpful to rely on when the literature does not provide any information.

Occasionally it is necessary to call the manufacturer concerning the availability or market release of a new agent. Although both

PharmIndex and *Facts and Comparisons* are useful in determining a new drug's availability, situations may arise when a newly released product has not been indexed in either of these references. When in doubt, the availability of a new product can always be determined by calling the manufacturer. The same procedure also applies for drug recalls, if this information cannot be found in reference sources.

It is helpful to contact the major drug manufacturers and ask to receive any information concerning the release of new drugs, new data on drugs that are already marketed and drug recalls. This information can prove invaluable to the pharmacist, and the pharmacist can contact the manufacturer either in writing or by telephone, using the "Manufacturers' Index" located in the front of the *Physicians' Desk Reference (PDR)*.

Investigational Drugs

Questions are sometimes received concerning the use of drugs for non-FDA approved indications, or on the use of investigational drugs not currently on the United States market. The recommendation of such agents for clinical use presents a dilemma to the pharmacist. Although many drugs are currently being used clinically for unapproved FDA indications, the final decision to use a drug must always be the physician's and this decision is independent of the pharmacist's input. The same applies for investigational drugs. Although the pharmacist may provide information on the use of the investigational drug, the physician must obtain the drug for use in his patients and follow the investigational drug protocol supplied by the company. The pharmacist should not hesitate to recommend therapy for non-FDA approved conditions if the therapy's effectiveness has been established by clinical studies. The following is an example of the type of question under discussion.

Request. (10/22/74) We have a patient with hemifacial spasms and would like to start therapy with carbamazepine (Tegretol®), on an empirical basis. As far as we know there is no FDA approval for using Tegretol® in this condition.

1. What is the liability of prescribing for non-FDA approved conditions?

2. How effective is Tegretol® in hemifacial spasms?

Response. 1. The only indications for carbamazepine (Tegretol®) use approved by the FDA are trigeminal neuralgia and glossopharyngeal neuralgia. However, there are many drugs used throughout the United States for conditions not approved by the FDA, carbamazepine being just one. For example, carbamazepine is definitely useful in tabes dorsalis and epilepsy and is used frequently and successfully for these conditions. The following is the position of the FDA on the use of approved drugs for unapproved conditions: "As the law now stands, therefore, FDA is charged with the responsibility for judging the safety and effectiveness of drugs and the truthfulness of their labeling. The physician is then responsible for making the final judgment as to which, if any, of the available drugs his patient will receive in the light of the information contained in their labeling and *other data* available to him."[3] However, once the drug is in the local pharmacy, the physician may vary the dosage and conditions for the use of the drug. "The physician should recognize that such use is investigational, and he should take account of the scientific principles, including the moral and ethical considerations, applicable to the safe use of investigational drugs in human patients."[3]

2. Only one study could be found on the use of carbamazepine (Tegretol®) in hemifacial spasms.[2] Another study used this drug in one patient with twitching and pain in the eye, but it was discontinued because of an allergic reaction.[1] Shaywitz[2] used carbamazepine 50 mg bid in an 8-year-old male with hemifacial spasms of several weeks duration. The spasms were characterized by intermittent, irregular muscle contractions involving the left orbicularis oculi. Within a month of initiating therapy, the facial movements had decreased to only a twitch and 2 weeks later they disappeared.

Carbamazepine reduces synaptic transmission in the spinal trigeminal nucleus. It is a very effective anticonvulsant and has actions similar to diphenylhydantoin; specifically, suppressing polysynaptic flexor reflexes with little effect on monosynaptic reflexes. It also decreases posttetanic potentiation of monosynaptic reflexes.[3] Based on these characteristics, it should be useful in hemifacial spasms. The drug has been used successfully in controlling paroxysmal symptoms in multiple sclerosis,[4] primary reading epilepsy with jaw jerking,[5] tonic seizures in multiple sclerosis patients[6] and focal epilepsy associated with hemifacial twitches of the lower face and lips.[7]

References

1. Krueger, W.: Uber Nebenwirkungen eines Azepinderivats (Tegretol®), *Med. Klin.* 61:674–676, 1966

2. Shaywitz, B.A.: Hemifacial Spasm in Childhood Treated with Carbamazepine, *Arch. Neurol.* 31:63, 1974

3. Crill, W.E.: Carbamazepine, *Ann. Intern. Med.* 79:844–847, 1973

4. Miley, C.E. and Forster, F.M.: Paroxysmal Signs and Symptoms in Multiple Sclerosis, *Neurology* 24:458–461, 1974

5. Gilligan, B.S.: Primary Reading Epilepsy. *Med. J. Aust.* 1:1025–1028, 1969

6. Kuroiwa, Y. and Shibasaki, H.: Carbamazepine for Tonic Seizure in Multiple Sclerosis. *Lancet* 1:116, 1967

7. Lerman, P. and Kivity-Ephraim, S.: Carbamazepine Sole Anticonvulsant for Focal Epilepsy of Childhood. *Epilepsia* 15:229–234, 1974

Formulating a Response

The Written Response

Most pharmacists, as well as drug information centers, respond to the majority of questions with verbal responses. Only a small percentage of the questions they receive are answered in a written format as an addition to the verbal reply. The written response is prepared for several reasons.

1. If the response took a considerable amount of time to research and prepare, the documentation of findings is important to avoid duplicating the same search if the question is asked again. Therefore, the response is considered valuable for future reference.

2. If the information was difficult to obtain or involved personal communications.

3. If the inquirer requests a written copy of the answer.

4. If the pharmacist has been asked to place the response in the patient's chart in the form of a consult.

In addition, it should be apparent that written responses or consults of merit depend on the documentation of fact and the personal experiences of the drug information pharmacist. Clinical experience must and should play a major role in the formulation of drug information responses. The pharmacist should feel an equal responsibility to the patients as to the individuals requesting information and, therefore, the pharmacist must and should do more than "just answer the question."

Written responses are useful for documenting the activities of the pharmacist, as well as the drug information service. They are also valuable in evaluating the effect of the service on patient care if adequate follow-up is obtained and added to the report. Here is an example of documenting the pharmacist's effectiveness with the use of a written report.

Request. (3/10/75) A 38-year-old female hyperthyroid patient has been on Tapazole® (methimazole) for 2 weeks (current dose 15 mg/day). She now presents with a generalized, giant, urticarial rash. Is this drug-induced? Will it subside with continued drug use?

Response. Skin rashes or urticaria are common forms of hypersensitivity reactions occurring with methimazole. These reactions occur early in therapy (first 3 weeks) and in as many as 5 percent of treated patients.[1,2] In recommended doses, the incidence of these reactions is probably greater than with propylthiouracil, but this may be due to the proportionately higher dosage rather than any inherent difference in toxicity. Skin rashes are usually not severe and may subside spontaneously while the patient is still taking the drug. However, if the reaction is generalized, a switch to a structurally dissimilar antithyroid agent (i.e., propylthiouracil) is advisable and usually successful.[3]

Wiberg and Nuttal[2] reported a variety of skin rashes occurring in 7 of 25 patients receiving high doses of methimazole. Four of these patients were later treated with propylthiouracil (PTU). Two patients had no toxic reactions to PTU, one developed a new but milder rash (therapy was continued without problems) and one had an identical reaction to PTU (urticarial reaction with marked dermatographia).

Horster et al.[4] successfully switched 6 patients to PTU after a previous allergic skin reaction to methimazole. The rash subsequently disappeared in all patients. In addition, a patient developing hepatitis with jaundice secondary to methimazole was successfully given PTU with resultant improvement in liver function. Thus, cross-sensitivity apparently does occur to some degree, but not in all patients.

If the reaction in this patient is considered severe, a switch to PTU is recommended. If the reaction remains severe, other forms of therapy should probably be considered (radioactive iodine, propranolol, reserpine, guanethidine, lithium carbonate).

References

1. Conn, W.F.: *Current Therapy*. W.B. Saunders Company, Philadelphia, 1975, p. 480

2. Wiberg, J.J. and Nuttal, F.Q.: Methimazole Toxicity from High Doses, *Ann. Intern. Med.* 77:414–416, 1972

3. Astwood, E.B.: Treating Hyperthyroidism, *Drug Ther.*: 92, 1973

4. Horster, F.A. et al.: Ergegniese der Behandlung von Hyperthyreosen mit Antithyreoidalen Substanzen, *Deutsch. Med. Wschr.* 90:377, 1965

5. Becker, C.E. et al.: Hepatitis from Methimazole During Adrenal Steroid Therapy for Malignant Exophthalmos, *J. Am. Med. Assoc.* 206:1787, 1968

Follow-up. Tapazole® was discontinued and therapy with PTU was instituted (3/12/75). As of 3/17/75, the rash has subsided without further sequelae.

Use of Tables and Graphs

When preparing a written as well as a verbal response to a drug information question which involves a large amount of data, it is often convenient to present the data in tabulated or graphical format. For the verbal response, this enables one to organize the data available for presentation over the phone more adequately, without recourse to fumbling through several articles or paragraphs summarizing the pertinent information. For the written response, this allows the data to be presented in a logical format and enables the inquirer to receive a summary of the subject in an easy-to-read fashion. Graphs may also be useful to present information, e.g., pharmacokinetic data. The use of tables in written responses can easily be adapted to any type of question, as demonstrated by the following adverse reaction example.

Request. (12/17/74) We have a patient with benign prostatic hypertrophy and hypertension. He developed hardening around the nipple area three months ago (unilateral). Biopsy was negative. This week, he developed hardening around the other nipple. Present medications are Aldactazide® (since February), two tablets daily; Aldomet®, 500 mg daily (6 months); and Valium®, 5 mg tid. Can Aldactazide® produce gynecomastia? If so, how long after initiation of therapy do symptoms appear?

Response. Spironolactone (in Aldactazide®) has been well documented to cause gynecomastia in males. [1-6] The effect is most clinically evident when higher doses are administered (400 mg/day),[7] but can occur with normal doses (100 mg/day).[5] Table 1 lists the pertinent findings in these reports:

Table 1. Spironolactone-Induced Gynecomastia: Analysis of Reports

AGE (YRS)	DIAGNOSIS	DOSE	DURATION	COMMENTS	REFERENCE
53	Nephrotic syndrome	400 mg/day	8 weeks	First report; subsided upon discontinuation	1
60	Cardiomy-opathy; CHF	100 mg q 6 hr	8 weeks	Swelling and discomfort in right breast after 4 weeks; bilateral after 8 weeks; remained unchanged despite halving the dose; remained on medication	2
56	Pitting edema —upper and lower extremities	*Course 1:* 100 mg tid (18.6 g total)	2 mos.	Pain and paresthesiae of both breasts; abated following drug discontinuation for 2 weeks	3
		Course 2: 300 mg/day 25 mg tid (14.7 g total)	1 mo. 4 mos.	Painful breasts; larger and firmer; decreased in size slowly after drug withdrawal	3
63	Nephrotic stage of chronic glomerulonephritis	300 mg/day 100 mg/day	2 weeks 2 years	Bilateral enlargement; drug continued despite gynecomastia	4
49	Hypertension	50 mg bid	4 mos.	Bilateral periareolar swelling of both breasts: resolved within 2 mos. after drug discontinuation	5

It is apparent that the gynecomastia can develop after only 2 weeks of therapy, or after as long as 2 years. Clark[6] reported a series of 12 patients treated with spironolactone. Four of the 7 male patients and none of the 5 women complained of hypertrophy of the breast. The alterations were invariably bilateral, characterized by pain, tenderness, lumpiness and enlargement, and occurred between 2 months and 13 months after initiation of therapy (50–100 mg/day). Disappearance of gynecomastia after withdrawal of spironolactone was not consistent and ranged from 41 days to 14 months.

Methyldopa (Aldomet®) has been reported to produce mammary hypertrophy and galactorrhea in females.[8,9] The drug reportedly has a propensity for producing gynecomastia in males,[10] but we found no cases of this nature in the literature.

The mechanism of spironolactone-induced gynecomastia is not clear. Spironolactone does have endocrine effects, due to its structural similarity to the steroid hormones, and antiandrogenic effects have been demonstrated in animals.[3,5,6] It must be assumed that these effects are, therefore, related to the steroid-like actions of the drug.

References

1. Smith, W.G.: Spironolactone and Gynaecomastia, Lancet 2:886, 1962

2. Williams, E.: Spironolactone and Gynaecomastia, Lancet 2:1113, 1962

3. Sussman, R.M.: Spironolactone and Gynaecomastia, Lancet 1:58, 1963

4. Mann, N.M.: Gynecomastia During Therapy with Spironolactone, J. Am. Med. Assoc. 184:778–780, 1963

5. Greenblatt, D.J. and Koch-Weser, J.: Gynecomastia and Impotence Complications of Spironolactone Therapy, J. Am. Med. Assoc. 223:82, 1973

6. Clark, E.: Spironolactone Therapy and Gynecomastia, J. Am. Med. Assoc. 193:157, 1965

7. Spark, R.F. and Melby, J.C.: Aldosteronism in Hypertension—The Spironolactone Response Test, Ann. Intern. Med. 49:685, 1968

8. Pettinger, W.A. et al.: Preliminary Communications: Lactation Due to Methyldopa. Br. Med. J. 1:1460, 1963.

9. Vaidya, R.A. et al.: Galactorrhea and Parkinson-like Syndrome: An Adverse Effect of Alpha-methyldopa, Metabolism 19:1068–1069, 1970

10. D'Arcy, P.F. and Griffin, J.P.: Iatrogenic Diseases. Oxford Medical Publications, New York, 1972, pp. 114–115

Follow-up. Spironolactone was discontinued. The gynecomastia has completely subsided over the past three months.

Conflicting Reports in the Literature

Conflicting literature reports are not an infrequent occurrence; in fact, matters of this nature represent an important area where the pharmacist skilled in providing drug information services can be of value. The ability to draw conclusions based upon a concensus of the literature is a necessary drug information skill in this situation. When confronted with conflicting therapeutic efficacy studies, the pharmacist must utilize the evaluative techniques described in Chapter Five to discriminate between well-designed studies and poorly designed studies, and draw his own conclusions in order to formulate an accurate, unbiased answer. The following response is based on inconclusive evidence and conflicting reports. This request was generated from a nursing home that heard of the value of gold leaf in the treatment of decubitus ulcers and was interested in employing this type of therapy for several patients in the home.

Request. (2/12/74) How effective is gold leaf for decubitus ulcers in elderly patients?

Response. Gallagher and Geschickter[1] successfully used gold leaf in 1964 in 10 patients to stop hemorrhaging from arteries, veins and capillaries in such varied regions as the cerebral and cerebellar cortex, the surface of the spinal cord and dura mater, muscle, spinal ligaments and periosteum. In the same year, Kanof[2] introduced gold leaf therapy for decubitus ulcers in nursing home patients with good results. This led to subsequent controlled studies to determine the true efficacy of gold leaf.

Wolf et al.[3] treated 20 decubitus ulcers in 11 patients with gold leaf. Three nontreated decubitus lesions served as controls. The lesions were saturated with 95 percent alcohol and covered with 4 to 8 layers of gold leaf, then a protective dressing was applied. This was repeated every 48 hours. Treatment was continued until healing was complete, the patient was no longer available, or resistance to therapy seemed evident. Sixteen out of 20 ulcers responded with an average decrease in area of 62 percent. Four did not respond at all, but this was probably due to excessive scar tissue or prolonged friction. The 3 control ulcers increased by an average of 96 percent. This study cannot be termed well controlled and the number of lesions treated is too few to evaluate the efficacy of gold leaf for a larger population.

Smith et al.[4] used gold leaf and other occlusive agents to treat 64 skin ulcers (17 decubitus) in 44 patients. These ulcers were treated with 8 to 12 layers of gold leaf and 95 percent ethanol, 3 with flexible collodion, 3 with aluminum foil and 3 with polyethylene film. Fifteen ulcers served as controls, with only ethanol being applied. Of the 40 ulcers treated with gold leaf, 33 were healed completely over an average period of 14 to 104 days, 4 showed 85 percent healing or greater, 1 showed 75 percent healing and 2 increased in size. In the control group 11 out of 15 ulcers healed completely over 18 to 54 days and 2 were 65 to 75 percent healed at the end of the observation period. Among the other occlusive agents used, flexible collodion is the only one that produced significant improvement; however, heavy crust formation was common. The response rate revealed that ulcers treated with gold leaf healed at the same rate or slower than the controls. Healing time was fifty-nine percent longer for ulcers treated with gold leaf than for controls.

These conflicting reports leave doubt as to the actual effectiveness of gold leaf in healing decubitus skin ulcers. It is proposed that gold leaf produces its effect by close adherence to the floor of skin ulcers, aided by the creation of a dielectric interface with ethyl alcohol. This close adherence maintains a moist wound surface to allow a more rapid epithelial migration.[2-4] However, the results of the study by Smith and associates suggest that an equivalent effect may be maintained by the use of adhesive, porous, dressing pads.[4]

References

1. Gallagher, J.P. and Geschickter, C.F.: The Use of Charged Gold Leaf in Surgery, *J. Am. Med. Assoc.* 189:928–933, 1964

2. Kanof, N.: Gold Leaf in Treatment of Cutaneous Ulcers, *J. Invest. Derm.* 43:441–442, 1964

3. Wolf, M. et al.: Gold-Leaf Treatment of Ischemic Skin Ulcers, *J. Am. Med. Assoc.* 196:693–696, 1966

4. Smith, K. W. et al.: A Comparison of Gold Leaf and Other Occlusive Therapy, *Arch. Derm.* 96:703–707, 1967

Disease State Background Knowledge

A large number of drug information requests involve the therapeutic use of drugs in the treatment of disease, or drugs as a cause of iatrogenic disease. A familiarity with the basic aspects of the disease state as it relates to the drugs enables the pharmacist to understand the circumstances surrounding the drug related problem better, and to provide a more useful response. Therefore, the pharmacist must have a fundamental knowledge of the disease state in question before attempting to provide a response or therapeutic recommendations. For example, if the pharmacist does not know the clinical manifestations of a given iatrogenic disease, an attempt to implicate a drug as the cause of that problem cannot be made.

Similarly, with the request: "We have a severely cirrhotic patient in congestive heart failure and would like to use furosemide. The patient is at present receiving thiazides and Aldactone®. Can the use of Lasix® with thiazides in this patient precipitate hepatic coma?" Unless the student has a knowledge of cirrhosis, congestive heart failure and hepatic coma, this question would be most difficult to answer. Standard medical textbooks such as *Harrison's Principles of Internal Medicine, Textbook of Medicine* (Beeson and McDermott) or *Current Medical Diagnosis and Treatment* (Krupp and Chatton) are useful for obtaining a disease state background.

Specific Problems

Problems with Synonyms, Indexing, and Medical Terminology

A common problem for students and pharmacists learning drug information skills is the use of incorrect indexing terms in the search for information. To complicate this, many secondary literature sources have their own method of indexing drugs, drug classes and disease states. For example, the *Iowa* System uses the American Hospital Formulary Service Classification System for indexing drugs, and the ICDA system for classifying diseases. *Index Medicus* uses medical subject headings (MeSH) from the National Library of Medicine. The *de Haen Drugs in Use* system uses its own disease classification. Foreign drugs present a similar problem. The student should look up synonyms for a particular disease state or foreign drug name if it is not found in the system searched. Lesch-Nyhan Syndrome, for example, may not be indexed as such, thus leading to an unproductive search for information, but a search under appropriate synonyms or other indexing possibilities may lead to a more productive search. For example, other possible sources of information on Lesch-Nyhan Syndrome would be found by searching under the headings mental retardation, hyperuricemia, spasticity and self-mutilation. Depending upon which indexing system is being used, original articles on Lesch-Nyhan syndrome could be found under any one of these terms.

Abbreviations can cause the same problem. For example, a question such as "What are the characteristics of nitrofurantoin-induced P.I.E.?" would not mean anything to the student unaware that P.I.E. means pulmonary infiltration with eosinophilia, a severe form of Loeffler's Syndrome. Therefore, students should consult medical dictionaries (e.g., *Stedman's Medical Dictionary*) or a textbook of medical synonyms and eponyms (Jablonski's *Illustrated Dictionary of Eponymic Syndromes and Diseases and their Synonyms*) to identify all indexing possibilities before initiating the search.

The News Media

On many occasions, calls will be received by the pharmacist regarding drug articles appearing in the lay press. The main source of these calls is the physician who has a patient in his office saying that he has read of a recent discovery which will cure his disease. The physician contacts the pharmacist to confirm or dispel beliefs about the efficacy of the agent in question. A newspaper frequently responsible for generating these types of questions is *The National Enquirer*, although other lay publications, including major newspapers, may publish information which is based upon speculative evidence or "testimonial" use of the drug. These publications are very seldom accurate, and rarely contain proof of the agent's efficacy.

Examples of controversies generated by these types of publication include laetrile as a cure for cancer, the use of clotrimazole in rheumatoid arthritis, the use of 5-HT and carbidopa to treat brain damage, the use of "wonder" drugs from Mexico to treat rheumatoid arthritis, hydrazine sulfate in cancer and the use of mixed respiratory vaccine and mixed influenza vaccine in rheumatoid arthritis. Since the pharmacist can expect calls of this nature, it may be useful to subscribe to one of these publications, e.g., *The National Enquirer*, in order to anticipate potential questions. As a general rule, a brief search of the literature will be helpful in dispelling these rumors. Sometimes it is of value to contact the local investigator, in order to obtain any unbiased data that might be available and perhaps information on clinical trials that are taking place to evaluate the purported therapeutic agent.

Teratogenicity

A very common question posed to the pharmacist concerns the adverse effects of drugs on the fetus. Answering such questions often presents a challenge, because of the lack of data in the literature on this subject and the fact that the data that are available are often incomplete. There are only a few textbooks which are helpful on this subject (see Chapter Four, table of references for adverse drug reactions), which means that original references pertaining to drugs used in pregnancy must be obtained.

When answering teratogenicity questions one must keep in mind that spontaneous malformations have a reported incidence between four and seven percent, and studies documenting the teratogenic effects of drugs must show an incidence significantly higher than four to seven percent to establish the drug as potentially or definitely teratogenic. Due to ethical considerations, prospective study is limited and most teratogenic studies dealing with large numbers of patients are retrospective. Another consideration is the risk vs. benefit in pregnancy. Although a drug may have teratogenic potential, discontinuation or avoidance of the drug in pregnancy may also seriously threaten the health of the mother and fetus. An example of this is the use of anticonvulsants in pregnancy. Phenytoin is documented as presenting a significant teratogenic risk when taken throughout pregnancy; however, many clinicians will agree that the absence of the drug during pregnancy in a patient with documented seizure activity is just as detrimental to the fetus should severe anoxia ensue secondary to seizures. Thus, anticonvulsants are recommended throughout pregnancy for patients with seizure disorders.

Before a conclusion can be drawn a thorough search of the literature as well as contact with the drug manufacturer is required, in order to obtain as much information as possible. The manufacturer may have a significant amount of unpublished data which could prove helpful. Several examples of questions regarding teratogenicity are presented in Chapter 8, together with methods for handling them. The following example describes a question on the use of mebendazole in pregnancy; no data is available and a conservative answer is given.

Request. (4/29/75) We have a 24-year-old female with pinworms (in a family of five) who is 9 weeks pregnant. We want to give her mebendazole (Vermox®). The package insert indicates the drug is contraindicated in pregnant women. Is Vermox® considered teratogenic?

Response. There are no published studies in animals or man reporting the teratogenic effects of mebendazole (Vermox®). Similarly, Ortho Pharmaceuticals has no data at present in this area.[1] Mebendazole does attain measurable plasma levels,[2] and because of its small molecular weight (about 295) is likely to cross the placental barrier.[3]

The FDA requires a contraindication statement regarding the use of the drug in pregnancy for all new drugs that have no proof of lack of teratogenicity. The only recommendation we can make at the present time is to avoid the use of the drug during the first trimester of pregnancy (specifically, between the 13th and 56th days of gestation) since the fetus is at the greatest risk during this time. If possible, of course, the drug should be avoided throughout pregnancy until teratogenic data becomes available.

References

1. Personal communication, Dr. Sargent, Medical Services Dept., Ortho Labs., Raritan, New Jersey
2. Brugmans, J. et al.: Mebendazole in Enterobiasis: Radiochemical and Pilot Clinical Study in 1,278 Subjects, *J. Am. Med. Assoc.* 217:313–316, 1971
3. Dentkos, S.: Passage of Drugs Across the Placenta. *Am. J. Hosp. Pharm.* 23:139–144, 1966

Self Evaluation Questions and Learning Examples on Situations and Problems in Providing Drug Information

7.1 Identify all areas and sources to be searched by the pharmacist in order for the statement "a complete search of the literature" to be made with assurance.

7.2 Identify what can be done if a "complete search" has been made and no data can be found.

7.3 Identify two sources of drug information outside the available literature resources and identify when they should be used.

7.4 Discuss how the pharmacist should formulate a response when there are (1) conflicting reports in the literature and (2) no data in the literature.

7.5 Discuss considerations that the pharmacist should be aware of when answering information requests concerning (1) the news media, (2) teratogenicity and (3) investigational drugs.

7.6 *Learning Examples.* Identify the classification type and missing background and history information, then prepare a written response using the recommended format for the following case examples. The key to these examples is in the Case Histories located in Chapter 8.

    a. How effective is respiratory UBA and influenza vaccine for rheumatoid arthritis?

    b. What are "crosstops"? Will they produce any adverse effects on the fetus?

    c. What is the recommended total daily dose of IV amphotericin B in cryptococcal meningitis? What toxic effects have been reported at this dose? What total doses and durations of therapy have been used?

    d. Is Salk vaccine still available in the United States? Who manufactures it?

    e. Can propranolol potentiate the hypoprothrombinemic effects of warfarin?

    f. Can blood transfusions lower alcohol blood levels from 100 mg/dl to 80 mg/dl?

    g. What is Ultralan®?

    h. Is Cotazym® still available?

    i. Why can't Valium® be mixed with other IV fluids? Is there any hazard in giving Valium® through IV tubing?

    j. Can clindamycin be safely mixed with Vitamin B complex (Solu-B, MVI®) in an IV infusion?

    k. How do you prepare a buffered ophthalmic solution of amphotericin B and nystatin?

    l. Can chronic exposure to carbon monoxide lead to parkinsonism?

8

The Systematic Approach Exemplified by Case Studies

163

Introduction

The case studies in this chapter are designed to provide the student with practical examples of questions that are commonly received by a drug information service. The format of each question follows the systematic approach outlined in this book, and thus will enable the student to visualize how this method can be used in practical situations. Appropriate comments are provided throughout, in order to emphasize certain aspects of drug information methodology and to review basic concepts that have been described elsewhere in this book.

Each request in this chapter is dated. This date represents the time the request was actually received by a drug information center. The dating of these requests is mentioned only because the information presented may not be up to date, e.g., information which would alter the response may have become available since the question was initially answered. Thus, these questions are not meant to actually teach concepts of therapeutics or clinical pharmacy practice, but are rather to exemplify the approach that should be used when answering drug information questions.

This chapter is divided into nine sections, as follows.

I. Drug Therapy and Efficacy Questions
    a. Clindamycin for *Clostridia* infections
    b. Drugs for *H. influenzae* meningitis resistant to ampicillin
    c. Mithramycin in Paget's disease
    d. Vaccines for arthritis
    e. Dextran 40 in thromboembolism prophylaxis
    f. Colchicine prophylaxis for gout

II. Adverse Reaction Questions
    a. Teratogenicity from Rubella vaccine
    b. Phenothiazine-induced leukopenia
    c. Nitrofurantoin-induced leukocytosis and fever
    d. Quinidine fever and rash
    e. Teratogenicity of "cross-tops"
    f. Physical dependence from propoxyphene

III. Drug Dosing Questions
    a. Cephalexin dosing in uremia

  b. Chloramphenicol for *H. influenzae* meningitis
  c. Amphotericin B in cryptococcal meningitis
  d. Betamethasone in the prevention of respiratory distress syndrome in newborns
  e. Carbenicillin in *Bacteroides* infection

IV. **Drug Identification Questions**
  a. Propirina®
  b. Ultralan®

V. **Drug Availability Questions**
  a. Sodium cellulose phosphate
  b. Salk vaccine
  c. Cotazym®

VI. **Drug Interaction**
  a. Antacids (Gelusil®) and anticonvulsants
  b. Propranolol and warfarin
  c. Methylphenidate and tricyclic antidepressants

VII. **Pharmacokinetics**
  a. Digoxin dosing
  b. Chloramphenicol (oral) in meningitis
  c. Ethanol kinetics

VIII. **Pharmaceutical Compatibility**
  a. Valium® in IV fluids
  b. Clindamycin and vitamin B complex (IV infusion)
  c. Amphotericin B and nystatin (ophthalmic solution)

IX. **Poisoning**
  a. Tri-Aqua® poisoning
  b. Dumb Cane plant poisoning
  c. Carbon Monoxide chronic toxicity

The self evaluation questions in Chapters 5, 6 and 7 are based upon the questions presented in this chapter, and it is hoped that the student will gain insight into the practical aspects of handling drug information questions by working up the self evaluation questions in these previous chapters properly.

Case Studies

I. Drug Therapy and Efficacy Questions

Is clindamycin considered the drug of choice for suspected *Clostridia* infections? (3/4/74)

Step I. Classification

1. *Request.* Concerns drug therapy; drug of choice
2. *Requestor.* Physician (internist)

Step II. Background Information

1. *Patient Data.* A 20-year-old female was admitted 3/1 with flank pain, left Bartholin's cyst and hematuria. She has a history of pelvic phlebitis and pulmonary embolism occurring two weeks previously.

2. *Laboratory Data.* Urinalysis (3/3): no bacterial growth. Urinalysis (3/4): a few gram-positive cocci. Left Bartholin's cyst drained 3/3—foul smelling pus. Cyst culture revealed gram-positive anaerobin rod (?*Clostridia*). Lab indicated that incorrect culture media was used for the isolation of *Bacteroides.*

3. *Medication History.* ASA 5 gr tid per 1 week. Current meds.—Cleocin® 300 mg po every 6 hours; Panwarfin® 5 mg daily.

Comment. The patient data in this case, as in most situations, changes the entire approach to the problem. Merely assuming that Cleocin® is effective or ineffective in this case would not answer the question satisfactorily. The physician is concerned about the overall treatment of the patient and not just one isolated piece of information. The pharmacist must approach the whole patient to formulate a usable response; in this case, any other information which may be helpful should be provided.

Step III. Systematic Search

Comment. Antibiotic therapy reference works should be checked first (Kucers and Bennett: *The Use of Antibiotics;* Kagan: *Antimicrobial Therapy*) to locate general information on anaerobic infections in the pelvic area. Then a search of the literature is required, in order to locate studies treating *Clostridia* and other possible anaerobes.

Stepwise search revealed the following references.

1. Johnstone, F.R. and Cockcroft W.H.: *Clostridium welchii* Resistance to Tetracycline, *Lancet* 1:660, 1968
2. Martin, W.J. et al.: In Vitro Antimicrobial Susceptibility of Anaerobic Bacteria Isolated from Clinical Specimens, *Antimicrob. Agents Chemother.* 1:148, 1972
3. DelBene, V. and Farrar, W.E.: Antimicrobial Therapy of Infections Due to Anaerobic Bacteria, *Sem. Drug Treat.* 2:295, 1972
4. Herrell, W.E.: Nonspore-Forming Anaerobic Bacteria Susceptible to Clindamycin, *Clin. Med.* 79:12, 1972
5. Thadepalli, H. et. al.: Anaerobic Infections of the Female Genital Tract: Bacteriologic and Therapeutic Aspects, *Am. J. Obstet. Gynecol.* 117:1034, 1973
6. Bartlett, J.G. et al.: Treatment of Anaerobic Infections with Lincomycin and Clindamycin, *New Engl. J. Med.* 287:1006, 1972
7. Kagan, B.M.: *Antimicrobial Therapy.* 2nd Ed., W. B. Saunders Co., Philadelphia, 1974

Step IV. Response

1. Although only a gram-positive anaerobic rod (possibly *Clostridia*) has been isolated at this point, the possible presence of *Bacteroides* and other anaerobes cannot be excluded, especially since the laboratory has indicated it did not use the correct culture media for the isolation of *Bacteroides*.

2. The antibiotic susceptibility of *Clostridium sp.* appears to have remained fairly consistent and penicillin G is still considered the drug of choice. Johnston and Cockcroft[1] found all of the 102 strains of *C. perfringens* tested to be sensitive to 0.15 units/ml of penicillin G. Similar findings were reported by Martin et al.[2] in 34 strains of *Clostridium perfringens* and *Clostridium sp.* Other agents shown to be effective are chloramphenicol, ampicillin, erythromycin and cephalothin.[3]

3. Clindamycin does not appear to be as effective in vitro against *Clostridia* as it is against other anaerobes, but Martin et al.[2] reported that 583 of 601 strains were sensitive to concentrations of 3.1 mcg/ml or less of clindamycin. Clindamycin was used in the treatment of 30 patients treated.[4] Thadepalli[5] treated 4 patients with mixed anaerobic infections of the genital tract (including *Clostridia*) with clindamycin. All patients responded satisfactorily. Of interest, there was one case in this group of infection of a Bartholin's gland. Culture of the gland abscess revealed only *Peptostreptococci.* Unfortunately, this case was not treated with clindamycin.

4. With this patient's current dosage regimen (300 mg po every 6 hours), serum levels of 3.6 mcg/ml will be reached 1 hour after oral administration, with levels falling to 1.1 mcg/ml at 6 hours. Depending on the susceptibility of *Clostridia* (or *Bacteroides*),

which is usually 0.1–3.1 mcg/ml (MIC), these levels may not be adequate, since occasional strains require higher serum levels. A dose of 450 mg every 6 hours is suggested, which will produce serum levels of 6.8 mcg/ml at 1 hour and 2.0 mcg/ml at 6 hours. Alternately, IM clindamycin may be considered. This will produce peak levels of 4–5 mcg/ml and 5.3 mcg/ml after doses of 300 mg and 450 mg, respectively, 2 to 4 hours after administration. At 12 hours, mean concentrations should be 1.2–0.16 mcg/ml and 2.5 mcg/ml, respectively.[6,7] *Bacteroides* is usually inhibited at concentrations of 3.1 mcg/ml or less, and these levels would cover this anaerobe if it is present.

    5. **Conclusion.** Clindamycin is a good choice for this infection, especially since other anaerobes may be present, although slightly higher doses (i.e., 450 mg) may be required. Penicillin G is more selective for *Clostridia* and may be used concomitantly. Besides *Bacteroides*, clindamycin will also be effective for most other anaerobes that are found on further cultures, as well as gram-positive cocci.

Step V. Follow-up

    On 3-3-75, clindamycin 300 mg q 6 hr was started; the dose was increased on 3-6-75 to 450 mg q 6 hr, per the DIS recommendation. Penicillin G, 1 million units q 6 hrs, was also started on 3-6-75. Bacterial cultures showed *Bacteroides, Clostridium perfringens* and *E. Coli* from the Bartholin's cyst. Urine cultures were negative.

    General improvement was first noted on 3-8-75, and this continued, with rapid improvement until discharge on 3-17-75 with take-home medications of Pen VK® 500 mg q 6 hr and Panwarfin® 5 mg daily.

How prevalent is ampicillin-resistant *Hemophilus influenzae* meningitis? Should chloramphenicol be considered the drug of choice for ampicillin-resistant *Hemophilus influenzae* meningitis? What other antibiotics have been used?

Step I. Classification

    1. Request. Drug Therapy
    2. Requestor. Physician (pediatrician)

Step II. Background Information

    1. Patient Data. An 18-month-old male (12 kg) with *H. influenzae* meningitis has not responded to ampicillin IV for three days.
    2. Medication History. At present: chloramphenicol

100 mg/kg/day IV. He had previously received a course of amoxicillin for *H. influenzae* otitis media.

Comment. This request arose mainly out of the concern of the physician over several recent cases of ampicillin-resistant *H. influenzae* meningitis; he was also very concerned about possible bone marrow depression from the use of chloramphenicol as a first line alternative.

In this case it is important to evaluate the available studies using other agents before a conclusion is drawn, and use of the original literature is mandatory. This is one instance where an accurate drug information response can change prescribing habits in the institution.

This request was received in 1974 when the increasing prevalence of ampicillin-resistance to *H. influenzae* was first being recognized. A search of the *Iowa Drug Information Service*, a *Medline* search and an *Index Medicus* search under meningitis is in order. It is important to obtain the most recent literature possible, as well as a review of resistant cases, to formulate a complete answer.

Step III. Systematic Search

Stepwise search produced the following references. All of the articles below were located with the use of *de Haen Drugs in Use* and the *Iowa Drug Information Service*.

1. Kandall, S.R. et al.: Ampicillin Failure in *H. Influenzae* Meningitis, *Clin. Pediatr.* 5:264–267, 1972
2. Ampicillin-Resistant *Hemophilus Influenzae* Meningitis—Maryland, Georgia, *Morbid. Mortal.* 23 (9):77–78, 1974
3. Tomeh, M.O. et al.: Ampicillin-Resistant *Haemophilus influenzae* Type B Infection. *J. Am. Med. Assoc.* 229:295–297, 1974
4. Khan, W. et al.: *Haemophilus Influenzae* Type B. Resistant to Ampicillin. A Report of Two Cases, *J. Am. Med. Assoc.* 229:298–301, 1974
5. Haltalin, K.C. et al.: Reevaluation of Ampicillin Therapy for *Hemophilus Influenzae* Meningitis, *Am. J. Dis. Child.* 122:328–336, 1971
6. *Haemophilus Influenzae* Meningitis Resistant to Ampicillin, *Med. Letter 16* (7):29, 1974
7. Walker, S.N. and Collins, C.C.: Failure of Cephaloridine in *Hemophilus Influenzae* Meningitis, *Am. J. Dis. Child.* 116:285, 1968.
8. Nelson, K.E. et al.: Treatment of *Hemophilus Influenzae* Meningitis: A Comparison of Chloramphenicol and Tetracycline, *J. Infect. Dis.* 125:459–465, 1972

Step IV. Response

1. Several cases of *Hemophilus influenzae* meningitis failing to respond to ampicillin have been reported in the literature since the first report in 1968.[1–5] This has undoubtedly resulted from the massive use of ampicillin in recent years. The mechanisms proposed for ampicillin resistance include poor penetration of ampicillin into the CSF, inadequate dosing of the drug, insufficient duration

of IV administration, and sequestration of organisms in sites inaccessible to the antibiotic.[3] Khan et al.[4] have proposed that the mechanism is due to the production of beta-lactamase by ampicillin-resistant strains. Substitution of chloramphenicol for ampicillin in these patients resulted in the prompt reduction of fever, with reduction in CSF white cell counts and negative cultures within a few days. Chloramphenicol is now considered the drug of choice for ampicillin-resistant strains of *H. influenzae* meningitis and should be given intravenously in doses of 100 mg/kg/day.[6]

2. Chloramphenicol was the drug of choice for *H. influenzae* meningitis long before ampicillin was available and it may supercede ampicillin as the drug of choice again if ampicillin-resistant strains continue to increase.[4] The main reason for using chloramphenicol in these patients is the very high CSF concentrations obtained with the drug (more than any other antibiotic).

3. Other antimicrobials used include gentamicin, sulfonamides, streptomycin, cephaloridine and tetracycline. However, none of these agents has proven superior to ampicillin or chloramphenicol and there have been no recent large-scale controlled studies using other antibiotics for this condition. Experience with gentamicin in *H. influenzae* meningitis is very limited. Streptomycin in combination with sulfonamides and penicillin was used in the past, but this has been superceded by the simplicity of therapy with ampicillin. Cephaloridine should not be used for the treatment of *H. influenzae* meningitis. The organism has been shown to be resistant to the agent in vitro and Walker and Collins[7] treated three cases with IV cephaloridine in doses of up to 600 mg/kg/day without obtaining a clinical cure.

4. Tetracycline, however, may have a place in the therapy of *H. influenzae* meningitis. Nelson et al.[8] compared tetracycline to chloramphenicol in 325 patients with *H. influenzae* meningitis. Patients (2 months to 6 years old) were given alternately tetracycline or chloramphenicol, in doses of 50 mg/kg/day IV. No significant differences between the two groups could be detected with respect to rates of mortality or morbidity, speed of defervescence, or rapidity of clinical recovery. However, the study was not double-blind, and if the recommended therapeutic doses of chloramphenicol had been used (100 mg/kg/day), the outcome may have been different. Chloramphenicol should still be considered the drug of choice for ampicillin resistant *H. influenzae* meningitis, but tetracycline is probably a good alternative if any evidence of bone marrow suppression appears during chloramphenicol therapy.

How effective is mithramycin in Paget's disease? How does it compare to other agents that have been used? (2/15/74)

Step I. Classification

1. *Request.* Drug therapy and drug efficacy
2. *Requestor.* Clinical pharmacist

Step II. Background Information

1. *Patient Data.* An 81-year-old female with disseminated Paget's disease. Probably involvement of skull area. Exhibiting symptoms of vertigo, headache, mental disturbances and weakness.
2. *Medications.* None at present. Considering mithramycin.

Comment. This is a "drug evaluation" type request. In general, these requests require the following types of information: review of proposed mechanism of action, evaluation of the available controlled clinical studies, comparison with other available agents, and a summary of the toxicity of expected adverse reactions. This request requires specific searching under mithramycin, which can be accomplished either through the *de Haen Drugs in Use System* or the *Iowa Drug Information System.* A *MEDLINE* search or quick review of *Current Contents* or *INPHARMA* may be useful in obtaining the most recent reports. *The Medical Letter on Drugs and Therapeutics* is also a good starting point for drug evaluation type questions. It enables a quick summary of the drug as well as pertinent references to be obtained and also provides an adequate style and format for the novice student.

Step III. Systematic Search

Stepwise search revealed the following references.

1. Ryan, W.G. et al.: Effects of Mithramycin on Paget's Disease of Bone, *Ann. Intern. Med. 70:*549–557, 1969
2. Ryan, W.G. et al.: Experiences in the Treatment of Paget's Disease of Bone with Mithramycin, *J. Am. Med. Assoc. 213:*1153–1157, 1970
3. Condon, J.R. et al.: Treatment of Paget's Disease of Bone with Mithramycin, *Br. Med. J. 1:*421–423, 1971
4. Evans, J.T. and Elias, E.G.: Mithramycin in Paget's Disease of Bone, *Clin. Res. 19:*714, 1971
5. Aitken, J.M. and Lindsay, R.: Mithramycin in Paget's Disease, *Lancet 1:*1177–1178, 1973
6. Mithramycin, *Med. Letter Drug. Ther. 12:*86–87, 1970
7. New Drugs for Treatment of Paget's Disease, *Med. Letter Drug. Ther. 14:*23–24, 1972
8. Kammerman, S.: New Modes of Therapy for Paget's Disease of Bone, *Am. J. Med. Sci. 263:*393–395, 1972
9. Barry, H.C.: Paget's Disease of Bone, *Practitioner 210:*340–350, 1973
10. Shai, F. et al.: The Clinical and Metabolic Effects of Porcine Calcitonin on Paget's Disease of Bone, *J. Clin. Invest. 50:*1927–1940, 1971
11. Woodhouse, J.H.Y. et al.: Human Calcitonin in the Treatment of Paget's Bone Disease, *Lancet 1:*1139–1143, 1971

12. Singer, F.R. and Bloch, K.J.: Antibodies and Clinical Resistance to Salmon Calcitonin, *Clin. Res.* 20:220, 1972

13. Haddad, J.G. and Caldwell, J.G.: Neutralizing Antibodies and Refractoriness to Porcine and Salmon Calcitonins, *Clin. Res.* 20:428, 1972

14. Smith, R. et al.: Diphosphonates and Paget's Disease of Bone, *Lancet* 1:945-947, 1971

15. Fennelly, J.J. and Groarke, J.F.: Effect of Actinomycin D on Paget's Disease of Bone, *Br. Med. J.* 1:423-426, 1971

16. Cordon, J.R.: Glucagon in the Treatment of Paget's Disease of Bone, *Br. Med. J.* 4:719-721, 1971

Step IV. Response

1. Clinical trials have shown mithramycin to be effective in Paget's disease.[1-5] It presumably acts by preventing excessive bone resorption through its cytotoxic effect on osteoclastic cells. This is supported by the fall in serum calcium following mithramycin therapy and the rapid fall in urinary hydroxyproline excretion, which reflects bone resorption rates. The gradual fall in serum alkaline phosphatase in these patients is attributed to a decrease in osteoblastic activity secondary to decreased bone resorption.[1,2] It has also been suggested that the beneficial effects of mithramycin are due to excess parathyroid hormone production as a result of the hypocalcemia produced.[3]

2. Ryan and associates[1,2] used mithramycin 15-25 mcg/kg/day by intravenous infusion in 15 severely pagetic patients. The duration of treatment for most patients was ten days. All patients responded well to treatment, as evidenced by symptomatic relief of pain and decreased serum alkaline phosphatase and urinary hydroxyproline levels. Of the 11 patients followed over 4 to 14 months, 6 had alkaline phosphatase values near to, or lower than, post-treatment levels. Condon et al.[3] administered mithramcyin in doses of 15 mcg/kg/day for 15 days to 3 patients, alternating 5 day treatment periods with 5 day drug-free periods. Significant relief of bone pain and a decrease in serum calcium, alkaline phosphatase and urinary hydroxyproline was obtained in all patients. A 2 to 8 month follow-up in these patients revealed no recurrence of pain. Evans and Ellis[4] achieved similar results in 10 patients using 25 mcg/kg/day IV infusions every 2 to 3 weeks. Complete pain relief was obtained in 7 patients, with partial relief in 2. More recently, Aitken and Lindsay[5] reported subjective improvement in 6 out of 10 patients receiving 15 mcg/kg intravenously on 5 to 15 occasions over 4 weeks.

3. Mithramycin is known to produce thrombocytopenia, hepatotoxicity, nephrotoxicity and hemorrhage by interfering with various clotting factors.[6] However, in the dosage and duration used in the above studies (usually 15-25 mcg/kg/day for 10 days), no

evidence of thrombocytopenia or clotting abnormalities was reported. Adverse effects that were observed included transient elevations in isocitric dehydrogenase,[1,2] microscopic hematuria with transient BUN elevations,[2,3] SGPT elevations,[5] decreased skin temperature and decreased cardiac output.[4] These effects were reversible upon discontinuation of therapy. Anorexia and nausea were reported, but were immediately relieved by discontinuing the drug for 2 or 3 days. Although toxic effects do not appear severe with these lower dosages, most authorities recommend that the drug be reserved for patients with extensive or rapidly progressive symptomatic disease.[1,2] The routine monitoring of renal, hematologic and liver function is mandatory with any dosage of mithramycin used.[7]

4. Other agents used in Paget's disease include ACTH, cortisone, high doses of aspirin, sodium fluoride (in doses of up to 120 mg/day), high calcium and phosphate diets, vitamin D, iodides, estrogens and androgens.[7-9] However, data are insufficient to evaluate the efficacy of any of these agents. Other drugs currently under investigation are calcitonin, the diphosphonates, actinomycin D and glucagon.

5. Porcine, salmon or human calcitonin acts mainly on osteoclasts to reduce bone resorption, and good results have been obtained in clinical studies.[10,11] There is evidence, however, that prolonged treatment results in hyperparathyroidism[7] and that porcine and salmon calcitonin can stimulate antibody formation to neutralize its own effect.[12,13] A decrease in effect has been reported over long periods of therapy with calcitonin. Disodium etidronate (a phosphonate) is relatively nontoxic, can be given orally, and has shown favorable results in a few patients.[1] It may act by retarding hydroxyapatite crystal dissolution.[8] Actinomycin D is reported to block the action of parathyroid hormone on bone and have a direct effect on osteoblasts and osteoclasts.[8] Good results were obtained in 3 of 4 patients receiving actinomycin D for 3 to 5 days,[15] but more clinical studies are needed to evaluate this agent. Glucagon, the better known of these agents, appears to act by stimulating the release of calcitonin from the thyroid gland. Clinical improvement was seen in 4 out of 4 patients receiving glucagon by IV infusion for 2-9 days.[16] All of these agents ultimately have the same mode of action, that is, inhibition of bone resorption, which results in decreased urinary hydroxyproline excretion and serum alkaline phosphatase values. More data is needed for comparison of these agents with mithramycin.

6. **Conclusion.** Both mithramycin and calcitonin have produced good results in uncontrolled studies of a small number of patients with Paget's disease. Calcitonin, however, is investigational in the United States and is not readily available. Mithramycin has

produced long-term remissions in several patients, without severe toxic effects, when used in doses of 15–25 mcg/kg/day. However, the drug should be reserved for patients with extensive disease and when it is used, constant monitoring of platelets, CBC, hepatic and renal function is essential.

How effective is respiratory UBA and influenza vaccine for rheumatoid arthritis? (7/23/76)

Step I. Classification

   1. *Request.* Drug efficacy
   2. *Requestor.* Physician (family practice)

Step II. Background Information

   1. *Patient Data.* none
   2. There have been several reports in the media and newspaper articles describing the use of mixed respiratory vaccine and influenza virus vaccine for arthritis. The most recent of these was reported in the *National Enquirer* in June, 1976. Several of my patients are demanding this treatment, based on these news items.
   Comment. This is a typical question generated by reports in the lay press. These types of questions are discussed in Chapter 7.

Step III. Systematic Search

   Comment. No references were found describing the efficacy of this therapy in the current literature, or from contacting the manufacturer. Contacting the original source of the information is usually helpful in formulating the response, but in this case, contacting the original source was of no help.

Step IV. Response

   1. There are no published reports, to our knowledge, using mixed respiratory vaccine and mixed influenza virus vaccine in arthritis. The only data available to us is a recent article in the *National Enquirer* reporting the use of mixed respiratory vaccine in combination with mixed influenza viral vaccine to treat chronic arthritis. This is a method developed by Bernard Bellew, M.D. in Desert Hot Springs, California. We contacted Dr. Bellew regarding this method, but he would give us no information and indicated that there were no published reports in this area. Although there are several testimonials indicating that this mixed vaccine therapy may be beneficial, there is no evidence to support these claims in the literature.

How effective is low molecular weight dextran (dextran 40) in the prevention of thromboembolism following fractures? (6/15/74)

Step I. Classification

1. *Request.* Drug efficacy
2. *Requestor.* Pharmacist (hospital)

Step II. Background Information

None. This was a straight-forward request regarding the efficacy of dextran 40, asked with no specific patient in mind. Many such drug-oriented questions are received by drug information centers and they should be afforded equal importance as a patient-related question, except that the latter type of question would receive a higher answering priority.

Step III. Systematic Search

Stepwise search revealed the following references.

1. Evarts, C.M. and Feil, E.J.: Prevention of Thromboembolic Disease After Elective Surgery of the Hip, *J. Bone Joint Surg.* 53A:1271–1280, 1971
2. Moreno, E.M.: The Use of Low Molecular Weight Dextran in Pulmonary Thromboembolism. *Arch. Inst. Carcoil. Mex.* 42:567–571, 1972
3. Salzman, E.W. et al.: Reduction in Venous Thromboembolism by Agents Affecting Platelet Function. *New Engl. J. Med.* 284:1287–1292, 1971
4. Langsjoen, P.H. and Murray, R.A.: Treatment of Postsurgical Thromboembolic Complications, *J. Am. Med. Assoc.* 218:855–860, 1971
5. Atik, M. et al.: Prevention of Fatal Pulmonary Embolism, *Surg. Gynecol. Obstet.* 130:403–413, 1970
6. Kimche, D. and Eisenkraft, S.: Prevention of Postoperative Thromboemboli by Combined Treatment with Low-Molecular Weight Dextran and a Proteinase Inhibitor, *Ann. Surg.* 173:164–172, 1971
7. Harris, W.H. et al.: Prevention of Venous Thromboembolism Following Total Hip Replacement. Warfarin vs. Dextran 40, *J. Am. Med. Assoc.* 220:1319–1322, 1972
8. Atik, M.: Dextran 40 and Dextran 70: A Review, *Arch. Surg.* 94:664–672, 1967
9. Rothermel, J.E. et al.: Dextran 40 and Thromboembolism in Total Hip Replacement Surgery, *Arch. Surg.* 160:135–137, 1973
10. Evarts, C.M.: Diagnosis and Treatment of Fat Embolism, *J. Am. Med. Assoc.* 194:157–159, 1965
11. Myhre, R. et al.: Dextran or Warfarin Sodium in the Prophylaxis of Venous Thrombosis, *Nord. Med.* 82:1534–1537, 1969
12. Ahlbert et al.: Dextran in Prophylaxis of Thrombosis in Fractures of the Hip, *Acta Chir. Scand.* 387:83–85, 1968

Step IV. Response

1. The incidence of thromboembolism associated with fractures of the hip, pelvis, or lower extremities was reviewed by Evarts and Feil.[1] In 8 studies involving 1,440 patients, thromboembolism

occurred in an average of 30 percent of cases. The reported incidence of thromboembolism after total hip replacement in 56 patients in their study was 53.6 percent. The use of dextrans to prevent these thromboembolic complications arose from a search for a safer and more reliable method than the use of anticoagulants. Anticoagulant prophylaxis has not been generally accepted because: it is not always fully effective; it may result in bleeding at the operative site and elsewhere; it is difficult to control and administer; and wound sepsis may increase. Dextrans are antithrombogenic agents which offer advantages by influencing platelet function without significantly altering the coagulation factors of the plasma proteins.[1] Dextrans produce their antithrombotic effect by decreasing platelet adhesiveness and aggregation, coating erythrocytes and endothelial walls, decreasing blood viscosity, reducing RBC rigidity, and hemodilution.[1,8]

2. Clinical dextran (dextran 70) has been used effectively to prevent thromboembolism in patients with fractures of the hip, pelvis and femur.[5,11,12] It is fairly well documented that dextran 40 and dextran 70 are equivalent in antithrombotic effect, and low molecular weight dextran should give the same clinical results as dextran 70.[5,8] Although some have reported better results with dextran 70, this may be due to a failure to infuse dextran 40 over a long enough period; dextran 40 is excreted more rapidly than dextran 70.[8] Dextran 70, although it has greater antithrombogenic potential, has been associated with a greater incidence of anaphylaxis, pulmonary edema and increased local bleeding in surgical wounds.[9] Low molecular weight dextran has been used successfully for treating fat embolism resulting from fractures of the femur.[10]

3. The high incidence of thromboembolism in patients undergoing hip surgery has provided an excellent opportunity to study the antithrombotic potential of dextran 40. Several studies have documented the effectiveness of dextran 40 in preventing thromboembolic disease in these patients.[1-4,6,7] Evarts and Feil[1] conducted a controlled study in 106 patients undergoing elective hip surgery. A total of 56 patients were untreated and 50 patients received either 500 or 1000 ml of dextran 40 on the day of surgery and then daily for 10–12 days. Using venography to detect the presence of thrombosis, 53.6 percent of the untreated patients were detected to have postoperative venous thrombosis, as compared to only 14 percent of the dextran 40 treated group. Langsjoen and Murray[4] reported that 7 out of 36 postsurgical orthopedic patients who served as controls developed thromboembolic complications; in 37 patients receiving dextran 40, none developed complications. One recent controlled study has reported no significant difference in detectable thromboembolism in patients receiving dextran 40

and control patients not receiving dextran 40. However, postsurgical venography or labelled fibrinogen uptake studies were not used to detect thromboembolism and conclusions as to the effectiveness of dextran should not be based on this study alone.[9]

4. To prevent thromboembolic complications, dextran 40 should be given shortly before, during and after operative procedures for hip replacement or fractures.[1,5] At least 500 ml should be started before induction of anesthesia and continued throughout surgery. Then 500 ml should be given in the postoperative period, followed by at least 500 ml daily for 7 days.[1]

5. Conclusion. Dextrans appear to have some benefit in the prevention of thromboembolism if used early enough. They are of no value in the treatment of thromboembolism. Further clinical trials using larger numbers of patients are needed. There is no evidence that dextran 40 is less effective than dextran 70.

Is colchicine of any real value in the prophylaxis of acute attacks of gout? Are any toxic effects associated with its long-term prophylactic use? (4/30/74)

Step 1. Classification

    1. Request. Drug therapy, efficacy
    2. Requestor. Clinical pharmacist

Step II. Background Information

    1. Patient Data. We have a patient with a history of gouty arthritis. She has remained symptom free on a regimen of probenecid and colchicine for eight years. I have found no references in recent literature indicating that colchicine is effective for gout prophylaxis.

Step III. Systematic Search

    Comment. From the nature of this question, and also because colchicine is a relatively old drug, the pharmacist should begin his search with earlier literature, using *Index Medicus,* since most of the work using colchicine for this purpose was probably done prior to 1960. A search of the *Iowa System* and the *de Haen Drugs in Use System* may be useful to screen for any recent references on this subject.

    Stepwise Search revealed the following references (all from *Index Medicus*).

      1. Cohen, A.: Gout, *Am. J. Med. Sci. 192:*488, 1936
      2. Talbott, J.H. and Coombs, F.S.: Metabolic Studies on Patients with Gout, *J. Am. Med. Assoc. 110:*1977–1982, 1938

3. Gutman, A.B. and Yu, T.F.: Gout, A Derangement of Purine Metabolism, *Adv. Intern. Med.* 5:227–302, 1952

4. Robinson, W.D.: Current Status of the Treatment of Gout, *J. Am. Med. Assoc.* 164:1670–1674, 1957

5. Rosenberg, E.F.: Gout: A Summary of Recent Developments in Therapy, *J. Am. Geriatr. Soc.* 2:229–239, 1954

6. Smyth, C.J. et al.: Treatment of Gout, *Arch. Intern. Med.* 97:783–792, 1956

7. Yu, T.F. and Gutman, A.B.: Efficacy of Colchicine Prophylaxis in Gout, *Ann. Intern. Med.* 55:179–192, 1961

8. Gutman, A.B.: Treatment of Primary Gout: The Present Status, *Arthritis Rheum.* 8:911–920, 1965

Step IV. Response

Several studies have documented the effectiveness of colchicine prophylaxis in gout, and have reported a remarkably low incidence of side effects even after long-term use. Cohen first described the use of colchicine as prophylaxis against acute gouty attacks in 1936.[1] He reported that the occurrence of acute gouty attacks was greatly reduced when colchicine was given in doses of 0.5 mg three times a day for one week in every four. Talbott and Coombs,[2] in 1938, modified the prophylactic regimen by giving small doses (0.0015 g) daily for two to three days each week to patients who had experienced more than two attacks of gout per year. Long-term use of colchicine was reported to be beneficial to the patients and without toxic effects. Gutman and Yu[3] used 0.5 to 1.5 mg colchicine nightly (or on alternate nights) in thirty-five patients for periods of six months to ten years. Acute attacks in thirty-one patients were virtually absent, or limited to occasional minor episodes readily aborted by an increased dosage of colchicine. No evidence of toxicity was reported and nine patients who were virtually incapacitated by gout were restored to partial or complete activity. The omission of colchicine for any length of time was often responsible for the early recurrence of acute gouty arthritis.

These sporadic reports of the prophylactic value of colchicine were encouraging and received much support,[4] but there was still skepticism regarding the efficacy and safety of this regimen, due to the lack of sufficient critical investigations.[5,6] Even up to the present, there have been no double-blind studies evaluating colchicine for this purpose. However, in 1961 Yu and Gutman[7] provided convincing evidence that colchicine given prophylactically was safe and effective in the prevention of gouty attacks. In this study, 208 gouty patients were given colchicine 0.5 to 2.0 mg daily for periods of two to more than ten years (mean, 5.4 years). All patients had a history of frequently recurring acute gouty arthritis. Of these, eighty-seven were nontophaceous and received colchicine alone throughout treatment. Thirty-two received only colchicine at first, but began to develop tophi after two to eight years and thus urico-suric agents were added to the regimen. Eighty-nine patients were intially tophaceous and were given colchicine and uricosuric drugs from the start. With respect to prevention of the occurrence of acute attacks, the results of prophylaxis were considered excellent in 153 cases (74 percent), satisfactory in forty-two cases (20 percent) and unsatisfactory in thirteen cases (six percent). There was no signifi-cant difference in the control of recurrent acute gouty arthritis between patients taking colchicine alone and those taking colchi-cine plus uricosurics. There were no untoward reactions to colchi-cine prophylaxis, except an initial hypersensitivity of the bowel occurring in four percent of the patients.

Since colchicine does not influence the metabolism or excre-tion of uric acid, it does not lower the hyperuricemia of gout or prevent the formation of tophaceous deposits (or reduce any al-ready present) and it is necessary to add uricosuric agents to the regimen (i.e., probenecid). Some feel that uricosuric therapy should be withheld until signs of early tophaceous deposits develop, since only a minority of gouty subjects will develop significant tophi, and then usually only after years of recurrent acute gouty arthritis.[7]

Conclusion. Although no controlled studies are available, colchicine prophylaxis of acute gouty attacks has been shown to be successful in a large number of patients treated over an extended period of time. This therapy has exhibited a very low incidence of side effects. Colchicine prophylaxis seems safe and effective for the majority of patients so treated.

II. Adverse Reaction Questions

What is the risk of teratogenicity with rubella vaccine? Is abortion indicated? (11/21/75)

Step I. Classification

1. *Request.* Adverse drug reaction; teratogenicity
2. *Requestor.* Physician (obstetrician)

Step II. Background Information

1. *Patient Data.* A 22-year-old female immunized with attenu-ated live rubella virus vaccine five days after conception. She was not aware of her pregnancy at the time of vaccination and her immune status is not known.
2. *Medications.* None
3. *Past Medical History.* Unremarkable

Comment. As discussed in Chapter 7, questions involving teratogenicity are relatively common in a drug information service, mainly because there is so little meaningful data available on this subject. Obtaining a careful background history is extremely important, especially the dose and duration of the suggested medication, other medications received and, most important, what stage of pregnancy was/is being confronted.

This question is especially difficult for two reasons: (1) rubella vaccine has a reputation as a potential teratogen and its inadvertent administration during pregnancy has already resulted in several therapeutic abortions, and (2) the pharmacist in this case is asked to make a decision regarding abortion. All questions of this nature must be handled conservatively and with as much objectivity as possible.

Step III. Systematic Search

Comment. Since rubella vaccine has been frequently implicated as a teratogen, finding literature on the subject should pose no problem. This is therefore one advantage to a question of this nature. It is worthwhile searching relevant drug monographs (*American Hospital Formulary Service, AMA Drug Evaluations*) as well as adverse drug reaction textbooks (Meyler's *Side Effects of Drugs,* Moser's *Diseases of Medical Progress*) to obtain perspective on the problem prior to searching the literature. This provides a "baseline" on current opinions and will give pertinent journal references, especially of the earlier literature. However, a decision should not be attempted until the original literature has been evaluated, for reasons explained earlier in this text. Texts such as *Drug Effects on the Fetus* and *Catalog of Teratogenic Agents* should also be consulted.

After these steps, a search of the *Iowa Drug Information System* and *de Haen Drugs in Use* will provide a useful compilation of references. No other systems (except *Current Contents* or *IN-PHARMA*) have to be searched, due to the relative frequency of articles published on this subject.

Stepwise search revealed the following references.

1. Chin, J. et al.: Avoidance of Rubella Immunization of Women During or Shortly Before Pregnancy, *J. Am. Med. Assoc. 215*:632, 1971
2. Levine, M.M. et al.: Live-Virus Vaccines in Pregnancy—Risks and Recommendations, *Lancet 2*:34, 1974
3. Mair, H.J. and Buchan, A.R.: Rubella Vaccination and Termination of Pregnancy. *Br. Med. J. 4*:271, 1972
4. Phillips, C.A. et al.: Intrauterine Rubella Infection Following Immunization with Rubella Vaccine, *J. Am. Med. Assoc. 213*:624, 1970
5. Larson, H.E. et al.: Inadvertent Rubella Virus Vaccination During Pregnancy, *New Engl. J. Med. 281*:870, 1971
6. Wyll, S. and Herrmann, K.: Inadvertent Rubella Vaccination of Pregnant Women, *J. Am. Med. Assoc. 225*:1472, 1973

7. Fleet, W. et al.: Fetal Consequences of Maternal Rubella Immunization, *J. Am. Med. Assoc.* 227:621, 1974

8. Wyll, S.: Risk of Rubella Vaccination During Pregnancy, *Obstet. Gynecol.* 38:641 (Letter) 1971

Step IV. Response

1. There are no well documented cases of teratogenicity secondary to the inadvertent administration of rubella vaccine during pregnancy; however, the possibility of embryopathy must be considered as a potential sequelae.[1-3] Accordingly, there is no well defined management of such cases. Some authors recommend therapeutic abortion, some do not. Fetal damage must be considered possible, but it is impossible to estimate the actual risk, as most of the cases of inadvertent administration of vaccine were followed by termination of pregnancy, or the prior immune status of the patient was not known.

2. Phillips et al.[4] reported a case of a 20-year-old seronegative woman who received rubella vaccine at 3 weeks gestation. Pregnancy was terminated at 8 weeks and rubella virus was isolated from decidua. The changes were considered similar to those seen in gestational rubella. Other studies have confirmed the presence of the virus in placental or fetal tissue following deliberate abortion.[5,6] However, whether such infections can result in congenital malformations is still unknown.

3. Wyll and Hermann[6] have indicated that rubella vaccine poses a definite hazard to the fetus, due to similarities between rubella vaccine and wild rubella infection of decidual, placental and fetal tissues. However, of 80 infants born to women in their study with unknown immune status who had received the vaccine in early pregnancy, all were clinically normal at birth. Fleet et al.[7] reported the results of 10 pregnancies (of unknown prior immune status) which were allowed to come to term following the inadvertent administration of rubella vaccine shortly before or during pregnancy. All infants appeared normal at birth and through follow-up. No viruses were isolated from oropharyngeal swab cultures in 9 infants. However, one case of fetal infection was reported, specifically, lenticular abnormalities typical of congenital rubella.

4. The Center for Disease Control has reviewed the findings of 148 vaccinated women, 131 of whom had an unknown immune status. Of these 131 women, 76 aborted (seven spontaneously) and 41 carried to term. The infants of the 41 mothers carrying to term were clinically normal at birth and rubella virus was not isolated from any products of conception.[8]

5. **Conclusion.** Inadvertent rubella vaccination shortly before or during early pregnancy definitely carries a risk of teratogenicity

due to its similarity to wild rubella virus. Seronegative women are obviously at greatest risk. However, there have been no reports of fetal abnormalities in the cases allowed to come to term. Since the immune status of the mother at the time of vaccination was usually unknown, interpretation of this data is of course difficult. However, at least 80 percent of the adult population has already acquired natural immunity to rubella; thus, the risk of vaccinating a seronegative pregnant female (who would be susceptible to viremia and fetal infection) is probably less than 20 percent. Based on this data, therapeutic abortion in this patient is not indicated. Many therapeutic abortions have been performed in rubella vaccinated pregnant women which, if not carried out, would probably have resulted in normal births.

Comment. A brief introduction to the problem should be followed by pertinent findings in the literature and a conclusion based upon these findings. Only primary reference sources should be used. Frequently, literature will be found after answering the initial response which will either fortify or dispute your original findings (as seen in the addendum below). The caller should be notified of these recent findings, if pertinent to the problem. In this case, a recent study in *The New England Journal of Medicine* supported our findings and the caller was notified of this new data.

Addendum. Modlin et al.[9] presented information regarding 343 women inadvertently given rubella vaccine shortly before or after conception. Of 172 infants carried to term, none had clinical or serologic evidence of rubella infection, including 38 infants of women known to be seronegative. Although there is a small risk of fetal infection, it appears to be very low (probably around 5 percent).

Reference

9. Modlin, J. et al.: Risk of Congenital Abnormality after Inadvertent Rubella Vaccination of Pregnant Women, *New Engl. J. Med. 294*:972, 1976

What are the characteristics of phenothiazine induced leukopenia? (3/28/74)

Step I. Classification

1. *Request.* Adverse drug reaction
2. *Requestor.* Physician (pediatrician)

Step II. Background Information

1. *Patient Data.* A 16-year-old Indian male admitted for hostile-aggressive behavior.

2. *Laboratory Data.* Values on admission:

	3/21	3/25
WBC	3700	4100
Segs.	58	36
Lymphs.	33	50
Eos.	2	5

Previous WBC count on 11/6/73:7200 with normal differential.
3. *Medications.* Received Thorazine® 25 mg qid from 2/7–2/25 (total 1.8 g). Currently receiving Dilantin® 100 mg tid, Mysoline® 250 mg tid, Mellaril® 100 mg bid (2/26 to present; as of 3/21/74, total dose of 4.8 g).
4. *History of grand mal seizures.* Currently being controlled well on Dilantin® and Mysoline®.

Comment. Again, it can be seen how important it is to obtain pertinent background information in order to assess the needs of the inquirer properly. For adverse reactions it is particularly important to obtain a history of all medications taken at present and during the past six months, the dose and duration of these medications, the onset of the suspected reaction (in this case leukopenia), a description of the reaction and any previous medical history in order to rule out drug-induced effects. Pertinent laboratory data are especially important, even if incomplete, as exemplified in this request.

Although anticonvulsants have been rarely associated with blood dyscrasias (leukopenia), the normal WBC count on 11/6/73 would tend to rule out these agents as etiologic factors. In addition, the dose and duration of phenothiazine therapy in this patient is consistent with doses reported in the literature to produce agranulocytosis.

Step III. Systematic Search

Comment. Pharmacology texts and drug monographs (*American Hospital Formulary Service; Martindale's, The Extra Pharmacopoeia,* etc.) should be consulted in order to obtain general information regarding the toxicity of phenothiazines on the bone marrow. This can serve as a "baseline" for previously reported adverse reactions. Information found in these texts, however, should not be used as the main source of response material. As mentioned previously, textbooks may provide statements from the literature which are not supported by adequate documentation. "Leukopenia" may be mentioned as an adverse effect, but the significance of the problem cannot be assessed until the original literature has been consulted and analyzed.

The next step is to consult adverse reaction textbooks (*Side*

Effects of Drugs, Diseases of Medical Progress, Drug Induced Diseases) to obtain a more detailed discussion of the reaction. Frequently, these texts will themselves serve as secondary references, since they will refer to the original literature. Frequently, the texts and references obtained from them will be the only sources that will be searched.

Other useful references for questions regarding phenothiazines and other psychotropic agents are *Psychotropic Drug Side Effects* (DiMascio and Shader) and *International Drug Therapy Newsletter* (F.Ayd, Editor). *Psychotropic Drug Side Effects* was one of the main references used to answer this question.

If incomplete or inadequate data was returned from the above mentioned sources, then a search of secondary literature sources becomes necessary. Usually, a search of the *de Haen Drugs in Use System* (under thioridazine) and the *Iowa Drug Information System* (under thioridazine, phenothiazines, or phenothiazines, toxicity) is all that is necessary. Most of the references listed below were obtained by this approach. It is important to remember that locating one good review article or recent case study will also provide additional useful references for the bibliography.

Stepwise research revealed the following references.

1. Pisciotta, A.: Drug-Induced Leukopenia and Aplastic Anemia, *Clin. Pharmacol. Ther. 12*:12–43, 1971
2. Erslev, A.J. and Wintrobe, M.M.: Detection and Prevention of Drug-Induced Blood Dyscrasias, *J. Am. Med. Assoc. 181*:114–119, 1962
3. Shader, R.I. and DiMascio, A.: *Psychotropic Drug Side Effects.* Williams and Wilkins Co., Baltimore, 1970, p. 165
4. Pisciotta, A.V.: Agranulocytosis Induced by Certain Phenothiazine Derivatives, *J. Am. Med. Assoc. 208*:1862–1868, 1969
5. Pisciotta, A.V. and Kaldahl, J.: Studies on Agranulocytosis: IV. Effects of Chlorpromazine on Nucleic Acid Synthesis of Bone Marrow Cells In Vitro, *Blood 20*:364–376, 1962
6. Baldwin, R.L. and Peters, J.E.: Hematologic Complications from Tranquilizers in Children, *South. Med. J. 61*:1072–1075, 1968
7. Pisciotta, A.: Hematological Safeguards During Treatment with the Phenothiazine Derivatives, *J. Am. Med. Assoc. 170*:662–664, 1959

Step IV. Response

1. Phenothiazines are undoubtedly the drugs most frequently associated with agranulocytosis.[1,2] Leukopenia occurs more frequently than agranulocytosis in patients treated with phenothiazines, with the majority of cases occurring in older individuals and most studies agreeing that it occurs more often in women than in men.[3] The reaction is characterized by a long latency period, ranging from 10 to 90 days from the beginning of treatment; about 90 percent of the cases occur within the first 8 weeks of treatment. It occurs very rarely with the short-term use of phenothiazines and is usually not seen until a cumulative dose of 5.0 g has been adminis-

tered.[4] The mechanism does not appear to be immunologic in nature. The long latency period suggests a toxic or metabolic mechanism, most likely involving interference with the bone marrow development of leukocytes.[1,4] This may be due to a direct toxic effect on the bone marrow, leading to inhibition of DNA synthesis in susceptible individuals.[5] A previously reacting patient may receive short-term therapy without it producing an immediate recurrence of agranulocytosis.[1,4]

2. Based on this patient's drug regimen, as well as the nature of phenothiazine-induced leukopenia, thioridazine is probably the etiologic agent producing the observed leukopenia. The findings of initial leukopenia followed by a gradual increase in white count in this patient are very similar to the findings of Baldwin and Peters.[6] They reported 9 cases of leukopenia out of 34 children (7–15 years old) treated with thioridazine 10 mg qid or 25 mg tid. Three patients exhibited a fall in leukocyte count of 1000 or more, 3 had a drop below 5000, 2 went as low as 4200, and 1 was as low as 2600. Leukopenia usually occurred within the first 8 weeks of treatment. In all the cases of leukopenia, white cell counts returned to *normal* levels in 20 days to 4 weeks *without* the discontinuation of the medication. There were no cases of agranulocytosis in the group.

3. The leukopenia in this patient appears to be following a similar course, as evidenced by the gradually increasing white count. At this point, there is no need to discontinue Mellaril® since agranulocytosis does not appear to be a problem. However, the patient should be observed closely for signs of infection, since when agranulocytosis occurs, the white count drops rapidly, reaching a low point in 2–5 days. Pisciotta[7] recommends that phenothiazines be stopped if the total leukocyte count drops below 3500, or if the total number of granulocytes represents less than 30 percent of the differential count. A leukocyte count between 3500 and 4000, with granulocytes between 30 and 50 percent, requires daily observation if the drug is to be continued. This is probably the best course to follow in this patient.

Step V. Follow-up

Mellaril was continued. The white blood count (WBC) on 3/30 was 6500 with 40 Segs. and 49 Lymphs. The white count has continued to climb. The patient was transferred to a mental health institution. No further data are available.

Can nitrofurantoin cause leukocytosis and fever? (5/22/74)

Step I. Classification

1. Request. Adverse drug reaction

2. *Requestor.* Pharmacist (outpatient clinic).

Step II. Background Information

1. *Medication Data.* A $1\frac{1}{2}$-year-old child (16 lbs) has been receiving nitrofurantoin 50 mg tid since 3/29/74 for urinary tract infection. The child has also been receiving phenobarbital 15 mg bid (reason not specified) and Fer-In-Sol® bid.

2. *Patient Data.* The patient has recently presented with symptoms of fever and anorexia with a leukocytosis (no lab data available).

Comment. The background information is limited in this case. As a general rule, the more nonspecific the patient data is, the less specific the response may be. However, it is possible to present a reasonable response with the data available in this request, as long as the duration of use of the drugs involved and the presenting symptoms are known.

Step III. Systematic Search

Comment. The search should begin with basic pharmacology texts and drug monographs, in order to elicit an overview of the toxicity of nitrofurantoin and the other agents the patient is receiving. Phenobarbital and iron can easily be ruled out as causative agents with these references. A search of the *Iowa* and/or *de Haen Drugs in Use System* will then be in order to locate the pertinent references.

Stepwise search revealed the following references.

1. Rosenow, E.C.: The Spectrum of Drug-Induced Pulmonary Disease, *Ann. Intern. Med.* 77:977–991, 1972

2. Larsson, S. et al.: Pulmonary Reaction to Nitrofurantoin, *Scand. J. Resp. Dis.* 54:105–110, 1973

3. Lubbers, P.: Chronic Interstitial Pneumonia with Pulmonary Fibrosis after Long-Term Nitrofurantoin Therapy, *Med. Klin.* 66:818–821, 1971

4. Muller, U. et al.: Pulmonary Hypersensitivity Reactions to Nitrofurantoin, *Schweiz. Med. Wschr.* 100:2206–2212, 1970

5. Wagner, A.: Chronic Interstitial Pneumonia with Pulmonary Fibrosis During Long-Term Nitrofurantoin Therapy, *Med. Klin.* 66:1808–1811, 1971

Step IV. Response

1. The only reactions of this type reported in the literature are those consistent with a pulmonary reaction to nitrofurantoin. There are two forms, one acute and one occurring after chronic use (3 months to 6 years).[1] The acute form has an onset of a few hours to 21 days after the start of therapy, and is characterized by cough, dyspnea, chills, fever, leukocytosis, eosinophilia, chest pain and

diffuse alveolar or alveolar-interstitial infiltrate seen on chest roentgenogram. The reaction resembles influenza.[1,2] The subacute or chronic form is usually not associated with fever, pleural effusion, or eosinophilia. The chest roentgenogram shows a diffuse interstitial fibrotic pattern.[1]

2. Although this is the typical pattern, several studies have observed leukocytosis, eosinophilia, weight loss and fever in the chronic form of the reaction to nitrofurantoin.[3-5] Most patients will improve upon withdrawal of the drug and the institution of corticosteroid therapy.[6]

3. However, the symptoms of anorexia in this patient may just be attributable to the gastrointestinal intolerance observed in patients taking nitrofurantoin, including those taking the macrocrystals (Macrodantin®). Fever and leukocytosis could be a manifestation of the infection being treated, or of some other infection as yet undiagnosed.

Can quinidine produce fever and rashes? (9/17/72)

Step I. Classification

1. *Request.* Adverse drug reaction
2. *Requestor.* Pharmacy student

Step II. Background Information

1. *Patient Data.* A 40-year-old male has received quinidine 200 mg daily for 1 week; the dose was increased to 400 mg for 3 days before the patient presented this morning with a maculopapular rash on the abdomen and a fever of 39.4°C (103°F).

2. *Medication Data.* Other medications: digoxin, Kaochlor®, Hydrodiuril®.

Comment. Many drug information services support clinical pharmacy teaching programs and pharmacy students are frequent users of the DIS in these institutions. This question is fairly straightforward and would not require much research.

Step III. Systematic Search

Comment. This question is a good example of how textbooks can be used as secondary literature sources. Moser's *Diseases of Medical Progress* discusses quinidine-induced rash and fever and also gives pertinent reference citations. Thus, the pharmacist can obtain the original article by referring only to this text. Other articles on the subject are undoubtedly available, but for the purpose of this request, one good case should suffice. Both references are cited in the report for completeness.

Stepwise search revealed the following references.

1. Moser, R.H.: *Diseases of Medical Progress*, 3rd edition, Charles C Thomas, Illinois, 1969, p. 102
2. Rose, O.A. et al.: Drug Fever Due to Quinidine, *New Engl. J. Med.* 248:96–98, 1953

Step IV. Response

1. The rash and fever exhibited by the patient is characteristic of a drug fever reaction to quinidine. Drug fever due to quinidine may occur with or without skin rashes.[1] Rose et al.[2] described the characteristics of drug fever associated with maculopapular eruptions due to quinidine in 3 patients. The temperature may reach as high as 40.6°C (105°F) without much discomfort to the patient. They also defined the criteria for identifying a drug fever reaction to quinidine. It usually occurs after regular drug administration over a period of 10 or more days, or after recent administration of the drug to a previously sensitized patient. There is a discrepancy between the relative well-being of the patient and the height of the fever. There is usually : concomitant allergic phenomena, especially an asymptomatic or slightly pruritic rash; the absence of any other cause for fever; and gradual defervescence over a period of 48 hours after the quinidine has been discontinued.

2. Although the reaction is rare, it could explain the symptoms in the patient. Procainamide should be substituted at this point to determine if quinidine is the causative agent.

Step V. Follow-up

Quinidine was discontinued and procainamide therapy was instituted. The rash and fever gradually subsided over the next few days.

What are "crosstops"? Will they produce any adverse effects on the fetus? (7/27/76)

Step I. Classification

1. *Request.* Drug identification; adverse drug reaction
2. *Requestor.* Physician (family practice).

Step II. Background Information

1. *Patient Data.* A 31-year-old female who is 8-weeks pregnant has been taking "crosstops" from a friend as an anorexic agent. She has taken 20 tablets over a 20 day period.

Comment. Not all questions presented to a DIS concern one specific item only; in fact, most questions are multifaceted in nature. These are easily handled by applying the systematic approach to each individual part of the question. In this case, we are dealing with a drug identification request as well as an adverse reaction. Each question is handled individually.

Step III. Systematic Search

Comment. "Cross-tops" is a slang term or street name. Drugs of this nature are usually not identifiable through standard drug identification sources. All drug information centers should maintain a file on "Drug Abuse," which contains a listing of slang names for street drugs. Another reference useful for this purpose is the *POISINDEX* system (Micromedex Incorporation), which includes slang names. The same reference sources mentioned in example IIA should be used to answer this question. Although there are several reports of teratogenic effects secondary to amphetamine use, the data is not conclusive enough to definitely implicate the drug. This is the case with most questions concerning teratogenicity. One important source of information should be the drug manufacturer. As mentioned earlier, most major drug manufacturers will have on file several cases of drug use during pregnancy which have not been reported in the clinical literature.

Stepwise search revealed the following references.

1. Schallock, M.: A Clinical Guide to Drug Usage During Pregnancy, *Alaska Med.* 16:37, 1974

2. Nora, J. et al.: Dextroamphetamine: A Possible Environmental Trigger in Cardiovascular Malformation, *Lancet* 1:1290, 1970

3. Levin, J.: Amphetamine Ingestion with Biliary Atresia, *J. Pediatr.* 79:130, 1971

4. Kasirsky, G. and Tansy, M.: Teratogenic Effects of Methamphetamine in Mice and Rabbits, *Teratology* 4:131, 1971

5. Personal communication with Abbott Labs., Medical Dept., Chicago, Illinois, (7/27/1976)

6. Briggs, G. et al.: Lack of Abnormalities in a Newborn Exposed to Amphetamine During Gestation. *Am. J. Dis. Child.* 129:249, 1975

Step IV. Response

1. "Cross-tops" is a street drug containing methamphetamine and sometimes other adulterants. Most "cross-tops" probably contain only methamphetamine.

2. The effects of methamphetamine and other amphetamine congeners on the fetus are not entirely clear in the literature. Several anecdotal reports of the possible teratogenicity of amphetamines have appeared in the literature, but a definite cause-effect relationship is at this point tenuous. Dextroamphetamine has been reported to cause transposition of the great vessels, congenital heart defects, biliary atresia, microcephaly and mental retardation, multiple abnormalities, exencephaly and possibly hyperbilirubinemia in

infants born to mothers taking the drug.[1-3] However, more confirmation is needed to ascertain the validity of these reports.

3. The teratogenic effects of methamphetamine have been reported in mice and rabbits.[4] The administration of large doses of intravenous methamphetamine hydrochloride was shown to produce several congenital anomalies, specifically exencephaly, cleft palate, microphthalmia, anophthalmia and cyclopia. However, this study cannot be definitely extrapolated to humans for obvious reasons. Abbott Laboratories (Desoxyn® brand of methamphetamine) reports one unpublished case of a mother who took 4–6 tablets of Desoxyn® (5 mg) daily for 2 months prior to, and for 3 months after, conception. The infant was born with deformities of the hands, fingers and toes. However, other reports from Abbott Laboratories of hundreds of patients using Desoxyn® for weight control during pregnancy report no real effects on the newborn infant when the drug was given throughout pregnancy.[5]

4. Briggs et al.[6] report a case of a woman with idiopathic narcolepsy who was treated with large doses of dextroamphetamine sulfate throughout pregnancy. The mother received 100 to 180 mg daily of Dexedrine® in addition to thyroglobulin 120 mg a day throughout pregnancy. A normal girl was delivered without signs of amphetamine intoxication, and after follow-up of 18 months, there was no evidence of toxic effects or malformations. The authors raised the question of placental transfer of dextroamphetamine and suggest that although the drug may enter the fetal circulation, it may not be in amounts substantial enough to be harmful to the fetus. More studies of this nature are necessary to determine the teratogenicity of amphetamine congeners.

5. **Conclusion.** Whether or not amphetamines are teratogenic remains unclear. Animal studies have reported a significant rate of congenital anomalies; however, there are also many reports of amphetamine ingestion during pregnancy without complications occurring in the infant. Malformations, if they do occur, probably occur at very high doses or when given for prolonged periods in the first trimester of pregnancy, but small to moderate doses (5 to 10 mg daily) will probably not produce any harmful effects. Since this patient received approximately 1 tablet daily for only 20 days, the chance of teratogenicity is very low; however, she should be advised against taking any amphetamine derivatives during pregnancy, as we do not have enough data available to make a complete evaluation of the teratogenic risk. One must also consider the fact that the spontaneous malformation rate is considered to be between 5 and 7 percent in the United States, and to prove that a drug is definitely teratogenic, one must demonstrate a malformation rate significantly higher than this level, which is often difficult to do.

What doses of Darvon Compound-65® are required to produce physical dependence? (6/17/75)

Step I. Classification

1. *Request.* Adverse Reaction
2. *Requestor.* Physician

Step II. Background Information

1. *Patient Data.* Thirty-eight-year-old female with chronic tension headaches has been taking Darvon Compound-65® for the past year. We are concerned about addiction and want to discontinue the drug.
2. *Medication History.* Darvon Compound-65®, eight capsules a day (520 mg propoxyphene).

Step III. Systematic Search

Stepwise search revealed the following references.

1. Miller, R. et al.: Propoxyphene Hydrochloride, *J. Am. Med. Assoc.* 213:996–1006, 1970
2. Fraser, H. and Isbell, H.: Pharmacology and Addiction Liability of dl-propoxyphene, *Bull. Narcot.* 12:9–14, 1970
3. Elson, A. and Domino, E.: Dextro-propoxyphene Addiction: Observations of a Case, *J. Am. Med. Assoc.* 183:482, 1963
4. Salguero, C. et al.: Propoxyphene Dependence, *J. Am. Med. Assoc.* 210:135–136, 1969
5. Wolfe, R. et al.: Propoxyphene (Darvon®) Addiction and Withdrawal Syndrome, *Ann. Intern. Med.* 70:773–776, 1969
6. Kane, F. and Norton, J.: Addiction to Propoxyphene. *J. Am. Med. Assoc.* 211:300, 1970
7. Claghorn, J. and Schoolar, J.: Propoxyphene Hydrochloride, A Drug of Abuse, *J. Am. Med. Assoc.* 196:1089, 1966
8. Daftery, A.: Naloxone Challenge in Propoxyphene Dependence, *New Engl. J. Med.* 291:979, 1974
9. Wesson, D. and Smith, D.: A Conceptual Approach to Detoxification, *J. Psychedelic Drugs* 6:167, 1974

Step IV. Response

Propoxyphene is very similar in structure to methadone and the drug can cause dependence of the morphine type when used chronically in high doses, but the potential for abuse is less than that for codeine.[1] Withdrawal symptoms are very similar to low-dose opiate withdrawal, and may include chills, diaphoresis, abdominal cramping, headache, lacrimation, myalgia, nausea and increased blood pressure. Propoxyphene can partially suppress abstinence symptoms in patients addicted to morphine when given in doses of 800 mg/day,[2] and propoxyphene napsylate is currently used to detoxify heroin addicts.

A thorough search of the literature reveals only a few well-documented cases of propoxyphene dependence.[3-7] Doses producing physical dependence in these studies range from 800 mg/day for several weeks to over 4 g/day for more than two years. Fraser and Isbell[2] reported five patients who received propoxyphene in doses of 600 to 825 mg daily for two months. Abrupt withdrawal produced only minimal abstinence symptoms. Very similar findings were reported by Elson and Domino.[3] Thus, it is apparent that daily doses of less than 750 to 800 mg are very unlikely to produce severe abstinence symptoms upon withdrawal. Claghorn and Schoolar[7] reported a case of acute organic brain syndrome and an acute psychotic episode secondary to propoxyphene-induced seizures in a female patient who had received fourteen capsules (910 mg) daily for five months prior to admission.

This patient is ingesting about eight capsules a day (500 mg propoxyphene) if the history is accurate, and although tolerance is developing to the drug, she is more likely to be psychologically dependent than physically dependent at this time. Gradual, or even abrupt, withdrawal should produce only mild or no abstinence symptoms at all. However, there is always the possibility that the patient is consuming more than the history indicates. In such a case, abrupt withdrawal would produce moderate to severe abstinence symptoms. Plasma levels would not be an accurate indicator of addiction liability in this patient (therapeutic levels are considered to be less than 200 mg/100 ml). Naloxone (Narcan®) challenge may be a valuable test in confirming her physical dependence to propoxyphene. Daftery[8] precipitated moderate withdrawal symptoms in two patients consuming large doses of Darvon Compound-65® for several years by injecting naloxone 0.8 mg IM. Withdrawal symptoms were noticeable within fifteen minutes following injection, and were similar in each patient—thus confirming definite physical addiction to the drug. Previous physical examination of the patients was unremarkable and there were no indications of adverse drug effects.

If the patient is suspected of taking larger doses of Darvon Compound-65®, or responds positively to the naloxone test, gradual drug withdrawal can be accommodated by substituting 50 mg of Darvon-N® (propoxyphene napsylate) for each 65 mg of propoxyphene hydrochloride. It is noted that withdrawal equivalency is not the same as analgesia. In this case, about 400 mg of Darvon-N® could be substituted for Darvon Compound-65® and given in daily divided doses. After the substitution, the napsylate can be withdrawn easily in step-wise increments of 50 mg/day.[9]

III. Drug Dosing

Will 1.0 g daily doses of Keflex® achieve adequate urinary concentrations in the presence of uremia? (2/13/76)

Step I. Classification

  1. Request. Drug dosing in renal failure
  2. Requestor. Physician

Step II. Background Information

  1. Patient Data. A 69-year-old (126 lb) female, admitted 2/11/76 for probable digitalis toxicity and acute urinary tract infection.
  2. Laboratory Data. C/S (2/11/76) revealed *Klebsiella* in the urine; MIC 12.5 mcg/ml (cephalexin). Creatinine clearance 10.6 ml/min, BUN 96 mg%, digoxin serum level 4.3 ng/ml (2/13).
  3. Medication History. Digoxin 0.25 mg/day since 1974; discontinued on 2/11/76. Presently receiving Keflex® 250 mg qid (1 dose given).

  Comment. For all questions regarding drug dosing in renal failure it is important to obtain the following information:
  1. age and weight of patient;
  2. diagnosis;
  3. culture and sensitivity (if available);
  4. renal function tests (creatinine clearance available); and
  5. route of administration of the drug.
Knowing these data, the pharmacist can (1) correlate clinical findings in the literature with those seen in the patient, and/or (2) calculate the correct dose of the drug, based upon renal function. In many cases, obtaining an accurate patient data base may result in further recommendations as to the therapeutic agent of choice, and thus also change the request to one of drug therapy.
  In this case, a knowledge of creatinine clearance is sufficient to formulate a reasonable response.

Step III. Systematic Search

  Comment. Several references are useful for drug dosing in renal failure. They include *Renal Function and Drug Action* (Reidenberg), *Clinical Use of Drugs in Renal Failure* (Anderson et al.) and Bennett, W.M. et al., *Ann. Intern. Med. 86:*754–783, 1977. Many questions can be answered with these references. However, to provide more specific information relating to a specific patient, it is helpful to obtain the original articles and the most recent studies in the area questioned.

Other reference sources for the use of antibiotics in renal insufficiency include, *The Use of Antibiotics* (Kucers), *Antimicrobial Therapy* (Kagan), *The Pharmacological Basis of Therapeutics* (Goodman and Gilman) and *The American Hospital Formulary Service.*

Stepwise research revealed the following references.

1. Giusti, D.: The Cephalosporins, *Drug Intell. Clin. Pharm.* 7:252, 1973
2. Kunin, C. and Finkelberg, Z.: Oral Cephalexin and Ampicillin: Antimicrobial Activity, Recovery in Urine, and Persistence in Blood of Uremic Patients, *Ann. Intern. Med.* 72:349, 1970

Step IV. Response

1. Certain requirements for antibiotic agents to be effective in the treatment of urinary infections in uremic patients are as follows. The ideal drug should be: nontoxic, even in high concentrations, so that no adjustment in dosage would be needed even if it were accumulated in the serum; excreted unchanged in the urine; and preferably cleared by tubular secretion, so that very high levels would be achieved in the urine. The only agents that approach these ideals are penicillins and cephalosporins.

2. Urinary recovery of cephalexin (Keflex®) is quite remarkable in normal patients and 97.6 percent of the drug is recovered within 6 hours of the first dose. In patients with uremia, urinary recovery of the drug is dependent upon renal function.[1,2] Kunin and Finkelberg[2] found that by using ordinary doses of cephalexin (500 mg q 8 hr) in uremic patients, accumulation is only modest and not associated with toxicity, yet therapeutic concentrations were achieved in the urine (although delayed by about one day) in uremic patients whose creatinine clearance exceeds 9 to 10 ml/min. Uremic subjects with a creatinine clearance of 9.2 or greater excreted the drug in the urine in proportion to their renal function. In one patient with a creatinine clearance of 9.2 ml/min, 10 percent of the dose was excreted in the urine within 6 hours of the last dose on the 8th day. One hundred percent of the drug was recovered in the 24 hours following the first dose in this patient. In severely uremic patients with creatinine clearances up to 2.5 ml/min or less, urinary concentrations are insufficient to inhibit antibacterial activity. Urine antibacterial activity studies revealed that good activity against most organisms (including *Klebsiella*) was obtained in uremic patients providing that their creatinine clearances exceeded 9 ml/min. Urinary antibacterial activity in uremic patients tended to increase as therapy was continued and remained present for at least 24 hours.

3. **Conclusion.** Cephalexin can be given to this patient in

doses of 500 mg every 8 hours without a large risk of accumulation or toxicity, including nephrotoxicity. Creatinine clearance should be monitored in the patient during cephalexin therapy at this dose, especially if the drug is given for a period of up to two weeks.

What is the maximum daily dose of chloramphenicol for *H. influenzae* meningitis? (11/26/76)

Step I. Classification

> 1. *Request.* Drug dosing (antibiotic)
> 2. *Requestor.* Physician

Step II. Background Information

> 1. *Patient Data.* A 20-year-old male (150 lb) was admitted with acute purulent sinusitis; *Haemophilus influenzae* meningitis is suspected.
> 2. *Laboratory Data On Admission.*

CSF—protein   154
CSF—glucose   55
CSF—WBC   765
CSF—RBC   33

CSF—gram-negative organism (C/S not returned).

> 3. *Medication History.* Chloramphenicol 4 g daily IV (started 11/26/74). Previous medications: Tylenol® prn, Sudafed® 1 bid, Colace® 50 mg in a.m., Nembutal® 100 mg hs, Afrin® Nasal Spray tid-qid, Valium® 10 mg qid.

Comment. This question appears relatively straight-forward. An accurate history should be elicited to rule out any drug-induced effects. Also, documentation of the organism is important in order to select the appropriate antibiotic. Although ampicillin is still considered the initial drug of choice for *H. influenzae* meningitis (in spite of reports of resistance), chloramphenicol produces the best CSF levels of any antibiotic and will eradicate most organisms, including *H. influenzae,* from the CSF.

Step III. Systematic Search

Comment. The best starting point is antibiotic textbooks such as Kagan's *Antimicrobial Therapy* in the section on meningitis. For completeness, however, a search of the recent literature will reveal several helpful studies which document the efficacy of chloramphenicol doses.

Systematic search revealed the following references.

1. Mathies, A.W. and Wehrle, P.F.: Management of Bacterial Meningitis in

Antimicrobial Therapy, 2nd edition. W.B. Saunders Company, Philadelphia, 1974, pp. 234–43.

2. Nelson, K.E. et al.: Treatment of *Hemophilus* Meningitis: A Comparison of Chloramphenicol and Tetracycline, *J. Infect. Dis. 125:459–65,* 1972

3. Schylkind, M.L. et al.; A Comparison of Ampicillin and Chloramphenicol Therapy in *Hemophilus influenzae* Meningitis, *Pediatrics 48:411–6,* 1971

4. Shackelford, P.G. et al.: Therapy of *Haemophilus Influenzae* Meningitis Reconsidered, *New Engl. J. Med. 287:634–8,* 1972

5. Eykyn, S. et al.: *Haemophilus influenzae* Meningitis in Adults, *Br. Med. J. 2:463,* 1974

Step IV. Response

1. The recommended dose of chloramphenicol for *H. influenzae* meningitis is 50–100 mg/kg/day in 4 divided doses for 10 days.[1-4] Some investigators recommend 100 mg/kg/day, but not to exceed 4 g daily.[1] Although the literature is not clear on this point, several studies have used 100 mg/kg/day in adults (without mentioning weight or daily gram doses) and it must be assumed that doses higher than 4 g daily have been used, i.e., 8 g/day in an 80 kg person.

2. A dose of 4 g is however adequate, based on the findings of Nelson et al.[2] Their results in treating *H. influenzae* meningitis in children with chloramphenicol 50 mg/kg/day compare favorably with results obtained from using 100 mg/kg/day or higher. Levels of chloramphenicol in CSF and blood are generally well above the MIC for *H. influenzae* with doses of 50 mg/kg/day. A dose of 50 mg/kg/day in this patient (150 lb) would be about 3.5 g. Eykin et al.[5] have recently reported excellent results using 3–4 g chloramphenicol daily in adults with *H. influenzae* meningitis.

What is the recommended total daily dose of amphotericin B in cryptococcal meningitis? What toxic effects have been reported at this dose? What total doses and durations of therapy have been used? (12/13/74)

Step I. Classification

1. *Request.* Dosing
2. *Requestor.* Physician

Step II. Background Information

1. *Patient Data.* We have a 41-year-old female with cryptococcal meningitis (determined from CSF culture). She is currently receiving amphotericin B 1 mg/kg/day IV (2 days).

2. We have found no clear-cut data regarding how much of the drug should be given in the majority of cases, and what toxicity we might expect. Some of our staff feel that 3 g is maximal to prevent undue toxicity.

Step III. Systematic Search

Comment. To provide an adequate response to this type of question it is useful to conduct a fairly complete search of the literature. This will reveal recovery rates at different dosages and data can be compared to arrive at a dose which has produced good clinical results. The use of a table is especially helpful in formulating responses of this nature. A search of drug monographs (*American Hospital Formulary Service, AMA Drug Evaluations*) will provide a background or summary of information on the subject, and antibiotic textbooks (*Use of Antibiotics, Antibiotics and Chemotherapy*) will present more specific data. Then a search of the *de Haen* or *Iowa* system under amphotericin B will reveal pertinent articles which can be used to formulate the response. *Index Medicus, Excerpta Medica Abstracts,* or *MEDLINE* could also be utilized. A search back to 1970 should be sufficient.

Stepwise search revealed the following references.

1. Kagan, B.M.: *Antimicrobial Therapy,* 2nd Ed., W.B. Saunders, Philadelphia, 1974, pp. 148–150

2. Newberry, W.M.: Drug Treatment of the Systemic Mycoses, *Sem. Drug Treat.,* 1972

3. *American Hospital Formulary Service,* Washington, D.C., (8:12.04 Amphotericin B)

4. Bindschadler, D.D. and Bennett, J.E.: A Pharmacologic Guide to the Clinical Use of Amphotericin B, *J. Infect. Dis. 120:*427, 1969

5. Bardana, E.J. et al.: Amphotericin B and Cryptococcal Infection. An Objective Method for the Evaluation of Treatment, *Arch. Intern. Med. 122:*517–520, 1968

6. Watkins, J.S. et al.: Two Cases of Cryptococcal Meningitis, One Treated with 5-Fluorocytosine, *Br. Med. J. 3:*29, 1969

7. Drutz, D.J. et al.: Hypokalemic Rhabdomyolysis and Myoglobinuria Following Amphotericin B Therapy, *J. Am. Med. Assoc. 211:*824–826, 1970

8. Gonyea, E.F.: Cisternal Puncture and Cryptococcal Meningitis *Arch. Neurol. 28:*200–201, 1973

9. Philpot, C.R. and Lo, D.: Cryptococcal Meningitis in Pregnancy, *Med. J. Aust. 2:*1005–1007, 1972

10. Dowell, A.R. et al.: Therapeutic Failure to 5-Fluorocytosine in a Patient with Cryptococcal Meningitis and Pneumonia, *J. Indiana Med. Assoc. 66:*1085–1088, 1973

11. Diamond, R.D. and Bennett, J.E.: Prognostic Factors in Cryptococcal Meningitis. A Study in 111 Cases, *Ann. Intern. Med. 80:*176–181, 1974

12. Sarosi, G.A. et al.: Amphotericin B in Cryptococcal Meningitis. Long-Term Results of Treatment, *Ann. Intern. Med. 71:*1079–1087, 1969

13. Cherry, J.D. et al.: Amphotericin B. Therapy in Children. A Review of the Literature and a Case Report. *J. Pediatr.* 75:1063–1069, 1969

Step IV. Response

1. There is no general agreement regarding the optimal daily dosage, total dosage, or duration of amphotericin B therapy for cryptococcal meningitis. Most sources recommend an initial test dose of 1 mg (in 250 ml dextrose), then increasing the dose in increments of 5–10 mg daily or every other day to the optimal dosage of 1 mg/kg/day IV, which is meant to achieve serum levels of 10 times the MIC.[1-3] Although some authorities recommend not exceeding 50 mg daily,[1] patients who do not respond to this optimal dose may be gradually increased to a maximum of 1.5 mg/kg/day, providing that no signs of toxicity develop.[3] 1.5 mg/kg/day is considered to be the maximum total daily dose. Bindschadler and Burnett[4] have shown that alternate day administration of amphotericin B, especially to patients showing clinical improvement or those on high dosage, may be as effective and better tolerated than daily administration.

2. Our review of the literature revealed that doses of 1 mg/kg/day or greater for prolonged periods has not been associated with an undue amount of toxicity. Pertinent findings from these studies are presented in Table 1. These results have shown that the frequency of infusions and daily dosage are controlled by the degree of azotemia, which is usually always present during IV administration. Creatinine clearance, serum creatinine and BUN frequently become abnormal, so that dosage must be reduced or the dosage interval increased. Hypokalemia frequently occurs, but can be controlled by oral supplementation. One case of hypokalemic rhabdomyolysis and myoglobinuria has been reported, but this complication is rare (see Table).

3. Two to four months is the usual treatment period, although some indicate that the total dosage of 2.5 g can be given over a 6 week period.[1] Although improvement may occur after one month of therapy, relapse may occur if the drug is discontinued too soon. The total dosage given also varies greatly. Total doses of 2–3 g have been recommended,[6,12] but generally, patients without underlying disease require a total of 3–5 g.[5] Doses as low as 300 mg have produced clinical cure,[11] but also doses as high as 5.7 g have been required.[12] Sarosi[12] reported death in a patient who had received 5 g for progressive meningitis. Bardana et al.[5] report that patients with underlying disease (i.e., diabetes) may require total doses of 5 to 8 g.

Table I. Amphotericin B Administration in Cyptococcal Meningitis

AGE	SEX	DOSE/ROUTE/ DURATION	RESULTS	ADVERSE EFFECTS	REFER- ENCE
34	M	50–87.5 mg/day (1.25 mg/kg/ day) IV; total: 3.185 g over 2½ mo.	Clinical improvement in 1 mo.; spinal fluid latex agglutination negative after 1 mo; cured	Elevated BUN and serum Cr (dose reduced to 50–75 mg/day)	5
64	F	.025–0.5 mg/day intrathecally (10 days), then IV 1 mg/kg/day (72 days); total: 3 g	Cured; clinical condition and CSF findings improved after 10 days	BUN elevation (41–75 mg%); persistent hypokalemia	6
24	M	0.05–0.75 mg/ day intrathecally (10 days), then IV to 350 mg total	Discontinued due to toxicity; treated successfully with flucytosine	BUN elevation to 90 mg%	6
20	M	25 mg/day (route not given; presumably IV) 75 days duration	Patient recovered despite toxicity; drug continued	Hypokalemic rhabdomyolysis and myoglobinuria (after 48 days); incomplete renal tubular acidosis; renal defect cleared in 1 year	7
45	M	2.6 g total IV over 11 weeks	Cured; no recurrence 4 years later	None	8
16 and 33	F	415 mg IV for 11 days (1); 1500 mg IV for 6 wks (1)	Clinical improvement in both, but one died	Nausea and vomiting (1); nausea and K+ losing nephropathy (1)	9

Table I. (*continued*)

AGE	SEX	DOSE/ROUTE/ DURATION	RESULTS	ADVERSE EFFECTS	REFER- ENCE
62	M	3 g IV over several weeks plus 0.5–1.0 mg intrathecally (20 doses)	CNS symptoms disappeared in 1 week; remained afebrile—the CSF protein remained elevated and cell count remained at 33 despite clinical improvement	None reported	10
Mean 45.1	69.4% Male	25–50 mg/day IV or 50 to 100 mg every other day; (35 pts received 1.5 mg intrathecally in addition to IV); total: 0.2–19.0 g	62 cured (total dose: 0.3–13.2 g); 18 cured with concomitant intrathecal injections	None reported	11
16– 71	M-19 F-12	42–5750 mg (total dose IV); 15 received intrathecal inj. in addition: 3–29 mg total dose	14 died (45%)—mortality due to meningitis in 12; 17 recovered (follow up 2–12 yrs); 4 have neurological sequelae	Not reported	12
4½	F	0.1 mg/kg initial IV, increased to 1.2 mg/kg/day for 13 days, then every 2 days for 5 wks	Cured; no growth of *C. neoformans* during therapy	BUN increased to 19.7 mg% (4th week); returned to normal after therapy	13

What is the recommended dosage of betamethasone to prevent respiratory depression in the newborn? (3/24/76)

Step I. Classification

1. *Request.* Drug dosage
2. *Requestor.* Pediatrician

Step II. Background Information

None. This question was not related to a specific patient.

Step III. Systematic Search

Stepwise search revealed the following references.

1. Fargier, P. et al.: Prevention of the Respiratory Distress Syndrome in Premature Infants. Value of Antepartum Glucocorticoid Therapy, *Nouv. Presse. Med.* 3:1595, 1974
2. Liggins, G. and Howie, R.: A Controlled Trial of Antepartum Glucocorticoid Treatment for Prevention of the Respiratory Distress Syndrome in Premature Infants, *Pediatrics* 50:515, 1972
3. Ballard, P. et al.: Glucocorticoid Levels in Maternal and Cord Serum after Prenatal Betamethasone Therapy to Prevent Respiratory Distress Syndrome, *J. Clin. Invest.* 56:1548, 1975

Step IV. Response

Fargier et al.[1] administered betamethasone phosphate 12 mg (6 mg phosphate and 6 mg acetate) IM daily for two days to thirty-five patients to prevent respiratory distress syndrome in premature infants. The incidence of hyaline membrane disease in the beta-methasone group was 4.4 percent, as compared to 20 percent in 375 controls.

Liggins and Howie[2] carried out a controlled trial of betamethasone therapy in 282 mothers in premature delivery to reduce the incidence of neonatal respiratory distress syndrome. Patients were given 12 mg betamethasone (6 mg betamethasone phosphate and 6 mg betamethasone acetate). Unless delivery had already occurred, a second injection was given twenty-four hours later. There were no deaths with hyaline membrane disease or intraventricular cerebral hemorrhage in infants of mothers who had received betamethasone for at least twenty-four hours prior to delivery. Respiratory distress syndrome occurred less often in betamethasone treated babies (9 percent) than in controls (26 percent), but the difference was confined to babies of under thirty-two weeks gestation who had been treated for at least twenty-four hours prior to delivery.

The safety of this mode of therapy has been evaluated by Ballard et al.[3] Serum corticosteroid levels were determined in twenty mothers and forty-three premature infants who received prenatal betamethasone for prevention of respiratory distress syndrome. A 12 mg IM injection of betamethasone (mixture of phosphate and acetate—Celestone Soluspan®) was administered and a second dose of betamethasone was administered twenty-four hours later if possible. Their findings indicated that serum corticosteroid levels from the injections can induce lung maturation, and that antenatal treatment with 12 mg betamethasone does not expose the human fetus to potentially harmful pharmacologic levels of steroid.

An IM injection of 12 mg betamethasone (Celestone Soluspan®) for one or possibly two days is considered safe and effective in preventing neonatal respiratory depression. This is especially significant if labor is delayed twenty-four hours after the injection.

IV. Drug Identification Questions

What is Propirina®? (9/21/76)

Step I. Classification

1. *Request.* Drug identification
2. *Requestor.* Physician

Step II. Background Information

1. *Patient Data.* This 42-year-old female has been taking Propirina®, two tablets three times a day for arthritis for one year. Recently, she returned from a trip to Mexicali, Mexico. She is also taking small, white, scored tablets for arthritis. She has developed hypertension in last few months (170/110) and we have started her on Hydrodiuril® 50 mg bid.

Comment. Very few drug identification questions are simple and straightforward; there is nearly always a secondary reason for the question being asked (poisoning, possible adverse reaction, etc.). This question is relatively simple, except for the fact that the patient is also receiving another unknown medication. This re-emphasizes the need for taking an adequate history, no matter how simple the question may seem.

Many patients with severe arthritis seek help from so-called "arthritis clinics" in Mexico. Corticosteroids, phenylbutazone, diazepam, indomethacin, etc., have been prescribed at these clinics in large amounts, which result in severe complications at a later date. Just identifying Propirina® in this case would not really help the caller to any great extent, since it contains only aspirin. The physician is mainly concerned if any of these agents could be inducing the hypertension in this patient. Thus, any information regarding the white, unscored tablets may be helpful.

Step III. Systematic Search

Comment. Most drug information centers subscribe to bulletins which keep them informed of drug misuse and abuse; specifically, the use of arthritis drugs in Mexican clinics. These can be invaluable in helping partially identify tablets such as the ones described in this question. In addition, the availability of a chemical laboratory to perform qualitative analysis on tablets such as these is very helpful. All centers should seek out laboratories of this nature for future use. Results of such analysis can be kept on file for future questions regarding the same type of tablet, etc. In this case, the most likely ingredient of this small white tablet is some corticosteroid which could be responsible for the recent development of hypertension in the patient. This is based on the analysis of several tablets of similar size from clinics in Mexicali, Mexico.

Propirina® is easily identified by using *Diccionario de Especialidades Farmaceuticas*, the Mexican equivalent of the *PDR*. If it were not a Mexican drug, then other sources such as *Pharmacological and Chemical Synonyms, Organic Medicaments and Their Synonyms, Index Nominum* and *USAN-10* should be starting points.

Systematic search revealed the following reference.

1. Rosenstein, E.: *Diccionario de Especialidades Farmaceuticas*, 23rd Ed., Drug Intelligence Publications, Hamilton Press, Inc., Hamilton, Illinois.

Step IV. Response

1. Propirina® (Chinoin Products, Mexico) contains 2-acetoxybenzoic acid 0.5 g per enteric coated tablet. This is acetylsalicylic acid (aspirin).

2. We suggest that the patient be further interviewed to ascertain if any other agents from Mexico are currently being taken. The white tablets she is taking could very well contain corticosteroids, which could in turn be responsible for this patient's hypertension. We have had several tablets analyzed qualitatively from a clinic in Mexicali, Mexico. Most of the small white tablets did contain a steroid. Please forward to us a sample of the white tablet so we can make a positive identification, or have it analyzed for corticosteroids.

Step V. Follow Up

Tablets were forwarded to DIC on September 29, 1976. The contents were analyzed and were found to include hydrocortisone. No further follow-up is available.

What is Ultralan®? (6/22/76)

Step I. Classification

1. *Request.* Drug Identification
2. *Requestor.* Physician

Step II. Background Information

1. *Patient Data.* I have a 38-year-old female arthritic in my office who is currently taking Ultralan® 20 mg tablets (Schering, Germany). Depending upon the appropriateness of the drug for the condition, I would like to prescribe a United States equivalent.

Step III. Systematic Search

Comment. Most drug identification questions can be easily handled by using the following reference sources: *Index Nominum, Martindale: The Extra Pharmacopoeia, Pharmacological and Clinical Synonyms, Organic Medicaments and Their Synonyms, USAN-10* and appropriate foreign compendia (e.g., *Diccionario de Especialidades Farmaceuticas*). Other reference sources which could be utilized include *Unlisted Drugs, de Haen Drugs and Research, Pharm Index,* and the *Iowa Drug Information System.* To locate a United States equivalent, the product should first be identified by using one of the above compendia. Then, an identical agent available in the United States or a similar agent available in the United States can be identified through using references such as *Facts and Comparisons, Pharm Index,* or *AMA Drug Evaluations.* In this particular case, the drug identified is not currently available in the United States. Therefore, it is necessary to compare the drug to a similar agent which is available in the United States. In this case, paramethasone is a reasonable equivalent.

The following references were utilized.

1. Jaspersen, H. (Ed.): *Index Nominum,* Drug Intelligence Publications, Inc., Hamilton, Illinois, 1975, p. 76
2. Rosenstein, E.: *Diccionario de Especialidades Farmaceuticas,* 23rd Ed. Drug Intelligence Publications, Inc., Hamilton, Illinois, 1974
3. Blacow, N. (Ed.): *Martindale: The Extra Pharmacopoeia,* 26th edition, The Pharmaceutical Press, London, 1972, pp. 520, 521

Step IV. Response

Ultralan® is a synthetic glucocorticoid called fluocortolone. It is available as tablets, ointments, cream, lotion and ophthalmic solution. It has a structure similar to that of paramethasone which, in turn, is very similar to dexamethasone. It is an anti-inflammatory with predominantly glucocorticoid effects, but does have some mineralocorticoid effects.[1-3]

The United States equivalent of Ultralan® would be Haldrone® (Lilly) or Stemex® (Syntex), which contain paramethasone acetate.

V. Drug Availability Questions

Is sodium cellulose phosphate available for clinical use? (2/20/76)

Step I. Classification

　　1. *Request.* Drug availability
　　2. *Requestor.* Physician

Step II. Background Information

　　1. *Patient Data.* We have a 48-year-old male with persistent hypercalcemia and nephrolithiasis. At a recent medical symposium, I heard of a drug called sodium cellulose phosphate, which is presumably effective for this condition.

Step III. Systematic Search

　　Comment. These references were both obtained through the *Iowa Drug Information System.*

　　Stepwise search revealed the following references.
　　1. Cellulose Phosphate. Investigational Drug Information, *Drug Intell. Clin. Pharm.* 8:182–183, 1974
　　2. Pak, C. et al.: Successful Treatment of Recurrent Nephrolithiasis (Calcium Stones) with Cellulose Phosphate, *New Engl. J. Med.* 290:175, 1974

Step IV. Response

　　Sodium cellulose phosphate (cellulose phosphate) is not currently available in the United States for clinical use. The drug is supplied by Whatman Biochemicals, Ltd., Springfield Mill, Maidstone, Kent, England. It is being sponsored as an investigational drug in the United States by the International Chemical and Nuclear Corporation.

　　The drug is currently being used to treat primary gastrointestinal hyperabsorption of calcium with resultant hypercalcemia and hypercalciuria and nephrolithiasis.[1,2] It is usually given in doses of 5 g two to three times daily with meals. When given orally, cellulose phosphate has been shown to bind calcium in the gut and increase its fecal excretion. Whereas cellulose phosphate may be absorbed, cellulose phosphate does not appear to alter serum phosphate or calcium, or calcium balance.[1] Pak et al.[2] treated sixteen patients with absorptive hypercalciuria and nephrolithiasis with cellulose phosphate 5 g two to three times daily. Urinary calcium decreased in all sixteen patients and urinary calcium saturation decreased in thirteen patients. Renal stone formation was significantly reduced in all patients treated. Treatment was well tolerated, and no serious side effects were reported.

Is Salk vaccine still available in the United States? Who manufactures it? (1/2/75)

Step I. Classification

1. *Request.* Drug availability
2. *Requestor.* Pharmacist (hospital)

Step II. Background information

None. This question was not related to a specific patient.

Step III. Systematic Search

Comment. References for drug availability questions parallel those used for drug identification in many respects. *Facts and Comparisons* is an excellent source, since the index will indicate if the drug has been withdrawn from the market. In addition, monthly updates are fairly reliable and include new agents that have been released for clinical use. *Pharm Index* is also a useful reference because of its "Products Pending" index. Monthly updates to the *Pharm Index* will include new drugs available on the United States market. If the drug is listed in the "Products Pending" index of *Pharm Index*, it is highly likely that the drug has not been approved for use in the United States and is still investigational. This is, however, not reliable in every case, as there is a one to two month lag period and the drug may have been released during this time. There are, in general, three other ways to determine if a drug is available on the United States market:

1. calling the manufacturer of the agent;
2. searching the recent medical and pharmaceutical journals for advertisements regarding the agent; and
3. making sure the Drug Information Center is on the mailing list of all major manufacturers, so that when new drugs are released it will be informed.

Other useful references for drug availability questions include the *American Drug Index* (however, not all drugs in *ADI* are marketed), *de Haen's Drugs in Use* (not all drugs in *de Haen's Drugs in Use* are marketed either, but it will usually indicate the manufacturer), *USAN-10, de Haen Drugs in Research* (most drugs here are investigational), *American Druggist Blue Book, Red Book* and *Physician's Desk Reference.*

In this case, a search of these references revealed that Salk vaccine had been taken off the market and the only source available at present is a company in Canada. More important than providing a source, is the reason why the vaccine was removed from the market, and this should be included in the answer.

Stepwise search revealed the following references.

1. Rotenburg, G.N.: *Compendium of Pharmaceuticals and Specialities (Canada)*, 8th Ed., 1973. Canadian Pharmaceutical Association, Toronto, Ontario, 1973

2. AMA Council on Drugs, *AMA Drug Evaluations*, 2nd Ed., Publishing Sciences Group., Acton, Mass., 1973, p. 872

Step IV. Response

Salk vaccine (formaldehyde-inactivated poliomyelitis vaccine) is no longer available in the United States. The Parke-Davis Company was the last manufacturer to supply the vaccine, but discontinued production in October, 1973. The only source we are aware of that still supplies the vaccine is Connaught Laboratories in Ontario, Canada (1755 Steeles Ave. W., Willowdale, Ontario; (416) 635-3613). The vaccine is supplied in 10 ml vials.[1]

Poliomyelitis (Salk) vaccine, however, is now used very infrequently due to the superiority of live, oral poliovirus (Sabin) vaccine. The live, oral vaccine is easier to administer, does not require booster doses and produces a long-lasting immunity resembling that induced by the natural infection. Repeated booster doses are required every two years with the Salk vaccine in order to maintain adequate antibody levels.[2]

Is Cotazym® still available? (9/9/75)

Step I. Classification

1. *Request.* Drug availability
2. *Requestor.* Physician (pediatrician)

Step II. Background Information

Several of my patients with cystic fibrosis have been having difficulty in obtaining Cotazym® tablets from local pharmacies. The pharmacists are indicating that there is a shortage of the drug. What is the reason for this shortage and what could we use as a reasonable alternative?

Comment. This is not a typical drug availability question, but this type of question is frequently asked of the Drug Information Center. Reference textbooks or other sources would not be helpful in answering this question, since the problem lies with the manufacturer.

Step III. Systematic Search

Comment. The only reliable way of obtaining data regarding this problem is to call the manufacturers. They will usually discuss reasons why the shortage has occurred and provide a possible source for obtaining emergency supplies of the drug.

Stepwise search revealed the following references.

1. Personal Communication with Organon Labs., West Orange, New Jersey
2. AMA Department of Drugs: *AMA Drug Evaluations*, 2nd Edition, Publishing Sciences Group, Inc., 1973, pp. 813–814

Step IV. Response

It appears that Organon Laboratories (Cotazym®) have been having a difficult time obtaining the pancreatic enzymes necessary for production of the drug. This has hopefully been alleviated and production and distribution should be normal in one to two months.[1] Until that time, local pharmacies may obtain Cotazym® directly from the Organon warehouse in North Hollywood, California, (213) 875-1752.

Reasonable alternatives for Cotazym® are pancreatin preparations which are derived from hog pancreas and contain amylase, trypsin, lipase and other constituents in varying amounts. Cotazym® (pancrelipase) has greater lipase activity as determined by in vitro measurements of the amount of glycerin (free fatty acids) formed by the digestion of fat. There are, however, no controlled clinical and metabolic studies to determine the relative efficacy of the various pancreatic enzyme preparations.[2] Doses of these products are (for children) 300-600 mg with each meal. The dose may be increased if no nausea, vomiting, or diarrhea occurs.

Table I. Reasonable Alternatives to Cotazym®

PREPARATION	AVAILABILITY
Pancreatin Triple Strength (Lilly)	Enseals, 0.32g (5 gr)
Panteric® (Parke-Davis)	Capsules, 0.32g (5 gr)
	Granules
	Enteric Tablets, 0.32g (5 gr)
Viokase® (Viobin) (Pancrelipase)	Tablets, 0.32g (5 gr)
	Powder

VI. Drug Interaction

Can Gelusil® increase the absorption of anticonvulsants, resulting in increased anticonvulsant serum levels? (7/1/74)

Step I. Classification

> 1. *Request.* Drug interaction
> 2. *Requestor.* Physician

Step II. Background Information

> 1. *Patient Data.* We have a 29-year-old patient who has been treated for generalized seizures with anticonvulsants for nine years. He has been adequately controlled during this time, with less than five seizures occurring per year. Last month the patient exhibited symptoms of phenytoin toxicity, consisting of nystagmus, slurred speech and ataxia. The levels of phenytoin and primidone (6-26-74) were 28 mcg/ml and 17 mcg/ml, respectively.
>
> 2. *Medication History.* Dilantin® 100 mg tid (since 1965), Mysoline® 500 mg bid and 250 mg at noon (since 1965). The patient has been suffering from constipation and dyspepsia, for which we added Gelusil 15 ml qid, Senokot® granules, Colace®, and Valium® 10 mg tid (all started on 4/3/74).
>
> **Comment.** Conducting a search of drug interaction references for interactions of antacids and anticonvulsants would not answer the question in this case. Again, the value of obtaining an accurate history is shown here. The pharmacist must consider all possible reasons that might explain the symptoms observed in the patient, and not just one isolated possibility, as presented by the physician in this case. For all drug interaction questions, the pharmacist must know the diagnosis, nature or symptoms of the suspected interaction, all drugs received by the patient in the last six months, the doses of the drug received and pertinent laboratory data, if available.

Step III. Systematic Search

> **Comment.** The most useful textbook source for drug interactions at present is *Drug Interactions* by Hansten. This provides a clinically useful discussion of each interaction, including the mechanism, clinical significance and management. Each interaction discussed is well referenced to the recent literature. The next most useful reference is *Evaluations of Drug Interactions* (American Pharmaceutical Association), which provides an entire monograph on a specific drug interaction. The limiting factors of both of these

references are that they do not include all interactions; however, the clinically significant interactions are usually included. Another reference source is *Handbook of Drug Interactions* by Hartshorn, which provides a discussion of the interactions in the text, together with tables of significant drug interactions. All of these texts are well referenced and will guide the user easily into the primary literature. Other reference sources which are useful as screening agents include *Cross Index Referenced Manual of Human Drug Interactions* (Sawyer), *Clinical Guide to Undesirable Drug Interactions and Interferences* (Garb), *A Manual of Adverse Drug Interactions* (D'Arcy), *Therapeutic Drug Interactions* (Cohen) and *Hazards of Medication* (Martin). *Drug Interactions I and II* (American Society of Hospital Pharmacists) is a useful secondary literature source for researching drug interaction questions. This is a spinoff publication from *International Pharmaceutical Abstracts* on Drug Interactions. *Interaction of Alcohol and Other Drugs* (Addiction Research Foundation) provides abstracts from the literature of adverse effects reported with drugs in combination with alcohol. *Drug Interactions—An Annotated Bibliography* is a compilation of abstracts on drug interactions produced by the de Haen Systems; it covers the period 1967 to 1971. *Clinalert* is a biweekly publication, which publishes abstracts, including drug interactions, from approximately 400 journals. Other systems which are very useful are the *de Haen Drugs In Use Systems, Iowa Drug Information Service* and *FDA Clinical Experience Abstracts.*

Systematic search revealed the following references.

1. Booker, H.E. et al.: A Clinical Study of Serum Primidone Levels, *Epilepsia* 11:395–402, 1970

2. Svensmark, O. et al.: 5,5-Diphenylhydantoin (Dilantin®) Blood Levels After Oral and Intravenous Doses in Man, *Acta. Pharmacol. Toxicol.* 16:331–346, 1960

3. Sparberg, M.: Diagnostically Confusing Complications of Diphenylhydantoin Therapy, *Ann. Intern. Med.* 59:914–930, 1968

4. Vajda, F. et al.: Interaction Between Phenytoin and Benzodiazepines, *Br. Med. J.* 1:346, 1971

5. Kutt, H. and McDowell, F.: Management of Epilepsy with Diphenylhydantoin Sodium, *J. Am. Med. Assoc.* 203:969–972, 1968

6. Treasure, T. and Toseland, P.A.: Hyperglycemia Due to Phenytoin Toxicity, *Arch. Dis. Child.* 46:563–564, 1971

Step IV. Response

Antacid preparations do not appear to have any significant effect on anticonvulsant blood levels. Both the primidone and diphenylhydantoin (DPH) serum levels are in the toxic range, and both drugs attribute to the observed toxic effect. Primidone serum levels above 10 mcg/ml have been associated with ataxia, nystagmus and drowsiness.[1] The dose this patient is receiving is considered high. One study has shown that doses of 1250 mg per day produced serum levels of 10–19 mcg/ml (mean 14.7), which is considered to be in the toxic range.[1] The reasons for the sudden elevation of DPH serum levels cannot be explained as easily. Svensmark et al.[2] reported DPH serum levels that were twice as high as expected in 19 of 29 institutionalized patients who had been taking DPH for years. Similar observations were made by Sparberg.[3] No apparent reason was given for these increases, but it is presumably due to variations in the metabolizing capabilities of microsomal enzymes responsible for DPH metabolism. Other reasons include, occasionally, excessive serum levels from a genetic inability to metabolize DPH, unintentional overdose, impaired metabolism from liver disease and interaction with other drugs. The latter reason seems more appropriate in this case.

Benzodiazepines (diazepam and chlordiazepoxide) have been reported to cause marked elevations in DPH plasma levels.[4] There have been reports of clinical intoxication associated with high DPH serum levels in patients receiving the combination[5] and one report of unexplained DPH toxicity in a patient receiving nitrazepam (similar to diazepam) in combination with DPH.[6] The interaction is most likely due to inhibition of DPH metabolism by the benzodiazepines. Although the interaction seems to be rare, it should be considered as a reason for the sudden toxicity in this patient.

In conclusion, the dose of primidone is probably too high, and should be reduced in this patient. The Valium® may be causing the excessive DPH serum levels and it should be discontinued if possible. If Valium® is to be continued, DPH serum levels should be monitored frequently and the patient observed for signs of DPH toxicity.

Can propranolol potentiate the hypoprothrombinemic effects of warfarin? (2/22/74)

Step I. Classification

1. *Request.* Drug interaction
2. *Requestor.* Clinical Pharmacist

Step II. Background Information

1. *Patient Data.* A 44-year-old male was admitted to the hospital for repeated bleeding episodes (nose, urinary tract). Prothrombin time on admission (2/22) was 24 seconds (control 11.55 seconds). The patient suffered a mild myocardial infarction in June, 1973, and has been stabilized on warfarin (Coumadin®) 5 mg daily since that time.

2. *Medication History.* Inderal® 60 mg daily since 1/4/74, Valium® 5 mg tid since 12/73, and Dalmane® 30 mg hs since 1/4/74. Coumadin® was started in June, 1973, and the patient is now stabilized on 5 mg/daily. The last prothrombin time (January 15, 1974) was 18 seconds (control eleven seconds).

Step III. Systematic Search

Comment. This is an example of a drug interaction which is not well documented in the literature. However, the interaction may be clinically significant in this one patient, despite the lack of reports of its frequency in the literature. Again, the systematic approach would be to seek drug interaction reference textbooks as well as drug monographs as screening agents. A search of secondary literature sources (*de Haen System, Iowa System, FDA Clinical Experience Abstracts*) under propranolol will reveal any studies documenting this particular interaction. It is important to correlate the findings in the case study with the patient in question, particularly with respect to dose and duration of therapy, other medications administered, reason for administering medication and other complicating diseases.

Systematic search revealed the following reference.

1. Neilson, G.H. and Seldon, W.A.: Propranolol in Angina Pectoris, *Med. J. Aust.* 56:856–857, 1969

Step IV. Response

To our knowledge, only one case of a propranolol-anticoagulant interaction has been reported. Neilson and Seldon[1] reported the efficacy of propranolol in the prevention of angina pectoris in twenty-five patients, three of whom were apparently well stabilized on oral phenindione therapy. The patients were given oral propranolol 160 mg/day for two weeks, followed by two weeks at 240 mg/day. Then either 240 mg propranolol or placebo was administered for a period of three weeks. Bleeding episodes occurred in all three patients stabilized on the anticoagulant, within six weeks of starting oral propranolol. In two of the patients, full hematological examination failed to reveal any reason for the bleeding.

The possibility of a drug interaction as a cause of bleeding in this patient cannot be ruled out, but there is not much evidence to document the occurrence of the interaction. It would be advisable to discontinue the propranolol in this patient and substitute another antiarrhythmic agent.

Step V. Follow-up

Procainamide (Pronestyl®) 350 mg qid was substituted for Inderal® on February 23, 1974. The patient's prothrombin time on February 23 was twenty-two seconds, and on February 24, 1974, nineteen seconds. The patient has not experienced any more bleeding episodes, although microscopic hematuria were present upon urinalysis on February 25, 1974. The patient was discharged on February 26, 1974, with a prothrombin time of 18.5 seconds.

How clinically significant is the methylphenidate-tricyclic antidepressant interaction? (4/2/74)

Step I. Classification

1. *Request.* Drug Interaction
2. *Requestor.* Clinical Pharmacist

Step II. Background Information

No background information. This request does not deal with a specific patient; this pharmacist has seen several patients on the combination and is curious as to whether the combination is rational or irrational, or if any significant interaction may occur.

Step III. Systematic Search

Stepwise search revealed the following references.

1. Garrettson, L.K. et al.: Methylphenidate Interaction with Both Anticonvulsants and Ethyl Biscoumacetate, *J. Am. Med. Assoc.* 207:2053–2056, 1969
2. Wharton, R.N. et al.: A Potential Clinical Use for Methylphenidate with Tricyclic Antidepressants, *Am. J. Psychiatry* 127:1619–1625, 1971
3. Perel, J.M. et al.: Inhibition of Imipramine Metabolism by Methylphenidate, *Fed. Proc.* 28:418, 1969
4. Zeidenberg, P. et al.: Clinical and Metabolic Studies with Imipramine in Man, *Am. J. Psychiatry* 127:1321–1326, 1971

Step IV. Response

Studies have shown that methylphenidate inhibits hepatic drug metabolizing enzymes[1] and elevates the blood levels of tricyclic antidepressants by inhibiting their hepatic metabolism.[2,3] The clinical significance of this interaction, however, appears to vary from patient to patient. Zeidenberg et al.[4] have shown that methylphenidate-induced increases in tricyclic antidepressant blood levels occur in some humans, but not others—suggesting individual sensitivity of drug metabolizing enzymes to methylphenidate.

Wharton et al.[2] reported improved clinical responses to imipramine in several patients when methylphenidate was added to the regimen. Seven patients with recurrent refractory psychotic depression were given imipramine, initially in doses ranging from

25–75 mg tid. When steady-state blood levels of imipramine were obtained (usually in three weeks), methylphenidate 10 mg bid was given and blood levels determined at least twice a week. The combination therapy was given for 10–21 days, then imipramine was continued alone for several more weeks with frequent plasma level determinations. Five of the seven patients on the combination therapy showed prompt and striking clinical remissions. In one patient, the imipramine blood levels rose from 310–320 mcg/l to 420 mcg/l while on methylphenidate. They indicated that methylphenidate given over a fourteen-day period may significantly inhibit the metabolism of imipramine, increase blood levels and enhance the desired therapeutic effect.

In conclusion, methylphenidate appears to elevate blood levels of tricyclic antidepressants in some patients. Patients receiving the combination should be observed for evidence of toxicity from the antidepressant, however, all that may be seen in an improvement in therapeutic response. Since both drugs act on the CNS, further studies are needed to determine if the improved clinical response is due to the increased antidepressant blood levels or to a direct effect of the methylphenidate. There have been no reports of tricyclic antidepressant toxicity from the combination.

VII. Pharmacokinetics

In a patient presenting with digitalis toxicity, how long must you wait before giving another dose? What should the new maintenance dose be? (7/18/75)

Step I. Classification

1. *Request.* Pharmacokinetics
2. *Requestor.* Physician

Step II. Background Information

1. *Patient Data.* A sixty-two-year-old male (70 kg) was admitted to the hospital today with symptoms of digitalis toxicity (anorexia, fatigue, vision disturbance and diarrhea). Occasional PVC's were noted upon physical examination.

2. *Medication.* Digoxin 0.25 mg every a.m. and 0.125 mg hs for CHF over the last 4 years. Hydrodiuril® 50 mg bid and KCl Elixir (10 percent) 15 ml tid for 4 years.

3. *Laboratory Data* Digoxin serum levels (7/16/75) were 3.6 ng/ml; serum creatinine 3.6 mg percent. The last dose of digoxin was taken on 7/16/75.

4. We want to restart digoxin at a safe dosage after abatement of the toxic symptoms.

Comment. This is a typical example of a question involving pharmacokinetic calculations. For all questions, including pharmacokinetics, the following background information is helpful:

1. age, sex and weight;
2. renal function tests;
3. hepatic function tests (if pertinent);
4. diagnosis;
5. drug serum levels or urine levels (if available); and
6. circumstances prompting the request.

Usually, as for many drug information questions, obtaining all the pertinent background data is difficult, and only a sketchy background may be available. However, the pharmacist should make every attempt to ascertain all pertinent data with regard to the patient.

Step III. Systematic Search

Comment. For patient-related questions, the primary literature is the best source of information. However, for initial pharmacokinetics data (normal blood levels, absorption, distribution, excretion), the use of general references is warranted (see Chapter 4).

Many pharmacokinetic questions involve dosing, and general references for drug dosing are also helpful.

The question presented here is relatively straight forward. A search of the *Iowa System* or *Index Medicus* will reveal pertinent original articles with sufficient data to make the necessary calculations.

Stepwise search revealed the following references.

1. Jelliffe, R.: An Improved Method of Digoxin Therapy, *Ann. Intern. Med.* 69:703, 1968
2. Clayton, B.: Reduction of Digitalis Glycoside Intoxication by Rational Dosing Procedures, *Am. J. Hosp. Pharm.* 31:855, 1974

Step IV. Response

Assuming this patient's renal function has not changed in the past 2 days, readjustment of digoxin dosage is calculated in the following manner.[1,2]

1. Calculate creatinine clearance.

$$Ccr = \frac{98 - 0.8 \, (age - 20)}{Cr}$$

$$Ccr = 18 \, ml/min$$

2. Calculate the percent daily doses.

$$\text{Percent lost per day} = 14\% + \frac{Ccr}{5} = 17.6\% = 18\%$$

3. Calculate total body glycoside level.

$$\frac{\text{Total Body Stores}}{(\text{Daily dose})(0.8)} = \frac{100\%}{\text{Daily losses (5)}};$$

$$X = 2000 \text{ mcg} = \text{Total Body Stores}$$

$$\text{Total Body Level} = \frac{2000 \text{ mcg}}{70 \text{ kg}} = 28 \text{ mcg/kg}$$

4. Desired body level for inotropic effect = 9–10 mcg/kg
   Desired Body Store = 10 mcg/kg × 70 kg = 0.7 mg

5. Using the percent daily losses, determine when the total body levels have dropped to half of the toxic levels:

Body level (mcg/kg)	Day 0	Day 1	Day 2	Day 3	Day 4
	28	23	19	16	13

Therefore, stop digoxin for ·4 days to allow the total body levels to drop accordingly.

6. Recalculate the maintenance dose needed to maintain 10 mcg/kg (0.7 mg):

$$\frac{0.7 \text{ mg}}{(x)(0.8)} = \frac{100\%}{18\%}; \ (x) = 0.16 \text{ mg/day}$$

7. Start the patient on 0.16 mg/day (elixir) 96 hours after the last dose to maintain peak body levels between 9–10 mcg/kg. Monitor the patient for toxicity or inadequate dosage and modify the dosage, based on changing renal status.

Are blood levels obtained from oral chloramphenicol palmitate lower than levels obtained with IV chloramphenicol? If so, what dose of the oral preparation must be given to produce equivalent blood levels? (8/27/74)

Step I. Classification

1. *Request.* Pharmacokinetics
2. *Requestor.* Physician

Step II. Background Information

1. *Patient Data.* A 21-month-old male (27 lb) with *Hemophilus Influenzae* meningitis resistant to ampicillin.

2. *Medication Data.* The patient has been receiving IV chloramphenicol 200 mg every 6 hours (for 3 days).

3. The patient is improving clinically, but we are having difficulty keeping the IV in the vein and would like to switch to oral therapy.

Step III. Systematic Search

Comment. The attainment of adequate blood or serum levels following absorption is a pharmacokinetics—type question, and in this case could mean treatment success or failure. Product formulations change with time, and it is always a good idea to check with the manufacturer for such data. The use of antibiotic textbooks and secondary literature sources (e.g., *de Haen Drugs in Use, Iowa System*) will reveal most other data necessary to answer the question.

Stepwise search revealed the following references.

1. Garrod, L.P. et al.: *Antibiotic and Chemotherapy,* 4th Ed., E. & S. Livingstone, London, 1973, pp. 137–138

2. Personal Communication: Dr. Pittelli, Medical Director and Dr. Hans, Pharmacologist, Parke-Davis Laboratories, Detroit, Michigan, 8/28/74

3. Snyder, M.J. and Woodward, T.E.: The Clinical Use of Chloramphenicol, *Med. Clin. North Am.* 54:1187, 1970

4. Kucers, A.: *The Use of Antibiotics—A Comprehensive Review With Clinical Emphasis,* Heinemann Medical Books, London, 1972, pp. 169–170

5. Weiss, C.F. et al.: Chloramphenicol in the Newborn Infant: A Physiologic Explanation of its Toxicity When Given in Excessive Doses, *New Engl. J. Med.* 262:787, 1960

6. Hodgman, J.E.: Chloramphenicol, *Pediatr. Clin. North Am.* 8:1027, 1961

7. Mossberg, H.O.: The Dosage of Chloromycetin Palmitate in Children, *Acta Pediatr.* 43:174, 1954

8. Yow, E.M. et al.: Chloromycetin Palmitate, *J. Pediatr.* 42:151, 1953

9. Aguiar, A.J. et al.: *J. Pharm. Sci.* 56:847, 1967

Step IV. Response

Chloramphenicol, when administered orally as the *base,* produces peak serum levels equivalent to, or higher than, those following IV administration.[1,2] After a 1 g oral dose, peak levels of 10–13 mcg/ml are obtained in about 2 hours, and sustained administration every 6 hours provides a cumulative effect with somewhat higher peak levels.[3,4] A 1 g IV dose of chloramphenicol sodium succinate produces similar blood levels, with peak levels occurring immediately. Blood levels obtained in children with an equivalent single oral or IV dose are of the same order.[4]

Chloramphenicol palmitate, however, must be hydrolyzed by pancreatic lipases in the duodenum before absorption occurs. Since absorption depends on hydrolysis, the rate of hydrolysis of the palmitate is a major factor in determining the ultimate blood levels achieved. Weiss, et al.[5] showed that the absorption of the palmitate

is slower in newborn infants because of a reduced rate of hydrolysis. Hodgman[6] reported that in older children, up to 50 percent of
an administered dose of palmitate may be lost in the feces and that
the dosage of the palmitate must be higher than that of the crystalline chloramphenicol base (100–200 mg/kg per day). This has also
been reported in earlier studies.[7,8] This slow hydrolysis, which
resulted in the lower blood levels reported by some investigators, is
due to the separate polymorphic states in which the palmitate can
exist. One crystalline form is substantially more hydrolyzed than
the other, and blood levels obtained are directly related to the
proportion of that form which is present in the preparation. This
was studied by Aguiar et al. in 1967.[9]

Being unable to support or refute the findings of Hodgman
and others with more recent clinical studies using chloramphenicol
palmitate, we contacted the Parke-Davis Company. They indicated
that subsequent to these reports, the less hydrolyzable polymorph
of the palmitate has been removed from the preparation and absorption of chloramphenicol from the palmitate is now complete
and reliable, producing blood levels equivalent to those following
IV administration.[2] These findings indicate that higher than normal
doses of the palmitate are not necessary. A dosage of 100 mg/kg/
day, in divided doses every 6 hours, will produce blood levels
equivalent to those obtained by IV or oral administration of the
base. Adequate CSF levels will be obtained, since concentrations of
chloramphenicol in the CSF reach levels as high as 50 percent of
those obtained in the blood and are well above the MIC for *H.
influenzae*.

In conclusion, oral chloramphenicol palmitate administration
to this patient will produce blood levels, and corresponding CSF
levels, equivalent to those obtained by the IV route when used in
doses of 100 mg/kg/day.

Step V. Follow up

Oral chloramphenicol palmitate 100 mg/kg/day was instituted. Within a few days the patient's condition improved, as
indicated by reduction of fever and reduction in CSF culture. He
recovered uneventfully, despite the appearance of a morbilliform
rash occurring after administration of the palmitate.

Can blood transfusions lower alcohol blood levels from 100 mg percent to 80 mg percent? (4/24/75)

Step I. Classification

1. *Request.* Pharmacokinetics
2. *Requestor.* Physician

Step II. Background Information

1. Patient Data. A twenty-eight-year-old male suffered severe trauma in an auto accident and required two units of whole blood. This blood alcohol level on admission was 100 mg percent.

2. Laboratory Data. The blood alcohol level drawn after transfusion was 80 mg percent.

Step III. Systematic Search

Comment. For this type of question, references are not always necessary, since all calculations can be made from known pharmacokinetic data on ethanol, which can be obtained from the textbooks listed in Chapter 4.

Step IV. Response

Ethanol distributes into the total body water (60 percent body weight). For a 70 kg man, the volume of distribution of ethanol would be 42 liters. If the minimum level required for intoxication is 100 mg percent, then the Ab for a 70 kg man would be:

$$Ab = CpVd \ (1 \ g/l)(42 \ l) = 42 \ g$$

The blood loss in this patient is approximately one liter and this is replaced by one liter of blood. Assuming the replacement liter is devoid of ethanol, then the ethanol loss would be 1 g.

Recalculating plasma concentration with the new figure for Ab, then:

$$Cp = \frac{Ab}{Vd} \text{ where new Ab} = 41 \ g$$

$$Cp = \frac{41 \ g}{42 \ l} = 0.98 \ g/l \text{ or 98 mg percent}$$

Therefore, at least from these calculations, it would be unlikely that the replacement of 1 l of blood would lower the ethanol plasma concentration from 100 mg percent to 80 mg percent for a 70 kg man. However, this assumes instantaneous replacement of the blood loss. Depending upon the time between loss and replacement of the blood, the amount metabolized by the body should also be accounted for. It is generally assumed that ethanol is metabolized by the body at a zero order rate equal to 10 g/hr. For the purposes of the example, assume the lag between blood loss and replacement for the above mentioned 70 kg man was one hour. Therefore:

$$Cp = \frac{41 \ g}{42 \ l} = 0.98 \ g/l \text{ or 98 mg percent}$$

$$\frac{31 \ g}{42 \ l} = 0.73 \ g/l \text{ or 73 mg percent}$$

In this case, the reduction of serum concentration, assuming normal metabolic processes, would be significant.

VIII. Pharmaceutical Compatibility

Why can't Valium® be mixed with other intravenous fluids? Is there any hazard in giving Valium® through IV tubing? (4/10/75)

Step I. Classification

1. *Request.* Pharmaceutical compatibility
2. *Requestor.* Nurse (intensive care unit)

Step II. Background Information

1. We have been routinely injecting Valium® through the tubing of an IV drip (using normal saline) in the Intensive Care Unit. We are concerned about possible precipitation of the drug and the associated complications, although we have seen no complications thus far.

Step III. Systematic Search

Comment. Questions involving intravenous incompatibilities are extremely difficult to answer because there are limited references in this area and the data are usually incomplete. In addition, the concentrations used in studies of incompatibilities usually differ from the concentrations that are used clinically, and it is difficult to extrapolate this data. Usually, however, enough information can be found to provide a fairly reasonable response to the incompatibility in question. At present, the most useful references for this purpose are the *Handbook of Injectable Drugs* (American Society of Hospital Pharmacists), *Guide to Parenteral Admixtures* (Cutter Laboratories) and *Intravenous Incompatibilities* (M. Cohen, University of Wisconsin). In addition, most drug information centers keep extensive files on recent articles discussing intravenous incompatibilities which represent the most up to date and complete information on the subject. Manufacturer's data is also helpful and should be kept on file. Other reference texts which are useful to screen IV compatibilities are the *American Hospital Formulary Service,* the intravenous incompatibilities table in *Hazards of Medication, Handbook of IV Additive Reviews—1971* (Drug Intelligence Publications), *Parenteral Drug Information Guide* (American Society of Hospital Pharmacists), and the chapter on IV incompatibilities in *Perspectives in Clinical Pharmacy* (Drug Intelligence Publications). Martindale's *Extra Pharmacopoeia* is useful in some cases of incompatibilities and cites studies from the literature. For some questions, such as the one presented here, a search of the literature (*Iowa System, de Haen System*) is useful for providing up-to-date references on the subject. For drugs that are used commonly, such as diazepam, there is usually a larger amount of literature, and, thus, several references dealing with the intravenous incompatibilities of the drug. For drugs used less, there is much less information in the literature on the subject and a search would probably not prove to be fruitful.

Stepwise search revealed the following references.

1. Trissel, L.A. et al.: *Parenteral Drug Information Guide*, American Society of Hospital Pharmacists, Washington, D.C., 1974, p. 58

2. Cohen, M.S.: *Intravenous Incompatibilities*, University of Wisconsin Medical Center, Madison, Wisconsin, 1971, p. 53

3. Juggo, W.J. et al.: Precipitation of Diazepam from Intravenous Preparations, *J. Am. Med. Assoc.* 225:176, 1973

4. Friedenberg, W. et al.: Intravenous Diazepam Administration, *J. Am. Med. Assoc.* 224:901, 1973

5. Dundee, J.W. and Haslett, W.H.: The Benzodiazepines, *Br. J. Anaesth.* 42:217, 1970

6. Langdon, D.E. et al.: Thrombophlebitis with Diazepam Used Intravenously, *J. Am. Med. Assoc.* 223:184–185, 1973

7. Cooner, J.A.: Diazepam Given Intravenously, *J. Am. Med. Assoc.* 224:1428, 1973

Step IV. Response

Diazepam is insoluble in water and aqueous solutions and should not be added to IV fluids.[1,2] This limited solubility has necessitated its formulation into a solution containing propylene glycol and alcohol, with sodium benzoate and benzoic acid as buffers and benzyl alcohol as a preservative. Dilution of this solvent system immediately results in a yellow-white precipitate of diazepam. If this solution is then acidified, a precipitate of benzoic acid may result and coprecipitate with the drug.[3,4] The maximal solubility of diazepam in normal saline is estimated at 0.3–0.4 mg/ml.[3] The clinical implications of using diluted diazepam infusions is twofold; (1) there is the probability that significant loss of potency of the diazepam would be observed, and (2) there is an increased risk of microemboli formation in the patient—possibly leading to thrombophlebitis and/or pulmonary embolism.

We are aware of no clinical "failures" in patients receiving IV infusions of diazepam in D_5W or NS, or in patients receiving the drug via IV tubing. Dundee and Haslett[5] discuss the use of infusions of diazepam-saline for various clinical situations. Although cloudiness appears in the solution, no loss of potency is observed. They recommend using IV infusions of the drug when prolonged IV therapy is necessary. This, of course, conflicts with the previous statements we have made and the technique is not recommended.

Thrombophlebitis has been reported as a complication of IV

diazepam use. Langdon et al.[6] have followed-up 590 of 651 patients who received IV diazepam and they report a 3.5 percent incidence of thrombophlebitis, which was protracted or severe in a few patients. It is not known whether the drug was given directly into the vein or via tubing, but if the drug was given through the tubing of an IV drip, it is possible that precipitation of the drug could have caused the thrombophlebitis.[3,4] Based on the flow rate of normal saline required to keep diazepam in solution during its addition to an IV infusion, it is highly likely that administration of the drug through the tubing of an IV drip will cause precipitation of the drug.[3] Although there is no conclusive evidence to show that flushing after IV diazepam prevents thrombophlebitis, most of the severe or protracted cases of thrombophlebitis in the series of Langdon et al. occurred in patients not receiving a flush.[6]

Conclusion. Administration of diazepam through the tubing of an IV drip can cause precipitation of the drug and result in thrombophlebitis. Two methods may be used to minimize this occurrence: (1) A scalp vein needle can be used to inject diazepam directly into the vein, and a filled syringe can be kept attached to the tubing for subsequent doses. (2) The tubing could be kept open with a solution, but the scalp vein needle should be flushed with the patient's own blood before more drug is injected.[4] Smaller veins should be avoided.[6] Cooner[7] reported an extremely low incidence of phlebitis. He used a 21-gauge scalp vein set connected to a bottle of saline and inserted a 5 ml syringe of Valium® through the rubber connector at the junction of the scalp vein tubing and the infusion tubing. Using a mosquito clamp to stop the flow of saline, the drug was injected in 2 mg increments, with the vein being flushed between doses with the saline.

Can clindamycin be safely mixed with vitamin B-complex (Solu-B®, MVI®) in an IV infusion? (3/18/75)

Step I. Classification

    1. Request. Pharmaceutical compatibility (IV admixture)
    2. Requestor. Pharmacist

Step II. Background Information

    None.

Step III. Systematic Search

    Comment. The literature on intravenous incompatibilities changes rapidly, and the most recent information should always be consulted. In this case, a search of available reference texts on IV incompatibilities revealed that this combination was incompatible. However, more recent evidence has indicated that the combination probably is compatible in certain concentrations. When a conflict such as this results, a call to the manufacturer is extremely helpful in ascertaining if any recent, and possibly unpublished, work has been done which supports the information found in the literature.

Stepwise search revealed the following references.

1. Trissel, L. et al.: *Parenteral Drug Information Guide*, American Society of Hospital Pharmacists, Inc., 1974

2. Personal communication with Mr. Woodward, Upjohn Co., Pharmaceutical Research Div., Kalamazoo, Michigan

Step IV. Response

Up to March, 1975, most IV incompatibility references and the manufacturer's product information indicated that clindamycin phosphate is incompatible with solutions containing B-complex vitamins. Recent information, however, indicates that this is not the case. One reference states that 600 mg Cleocin® phosphate may be added to Solu-B® in D_5W if the solution is used within 7 hours.[1]

The pharmaceutical research unit at Upjohn Co. has recently studied the compatibility of this combination and reports that Cleocin® phosphate and B-complex vitamins are now considered an acceptable mixture. Solu-B-Forte® (10 ml) with 600 mg Cleocin® phosphate in 1000 ml D_5W was found to be stable for 24 hours at room temperature.[2] This corrected information will appear on the May, 1975 package insert for Cleocin® phosphate.

How do you prepare buffered ophthalmic solutions of amphotericin B and nystatin? (1/1/75)

Step I. Classification

1. *Request.* Pharmaceutical compatibility (extemporaneous)
2. *Requestor.* Pharmacist (hospital)

Step II. Background Information

1. *Patient Data.* A 42-year-old male has fungal keratitis. The physician is considering the use of topical ocular amphotericin B (10 mg/ml) or nystatin 100,000 units/ml.

Step III. Systematic Search

Comment. This type of question falls into the pharmaceutical compatibility classification, although it deals mainly with compounding. Useful references for this type of request are Remington's *Pharmaceutical Sciences*, Husa's *Dispensing of Medication* and

Martindale's Extra Pharmacopoeia. In addition, for ophthalmic preparations, Havener's *Ocular Pharmacology* is most useful. A search of the literature via the *Iowa System* or *de Haen System* will usually provide pertinent references. For example, a study will be found using topical amphotericin B or nystatin for a fungal keratitis. Upon retrieving the original reference, a discussion of the preparation of these drugs for ocular installation is usually included. This applies to other types of questions as well, including the mixing of drugs for intravenous infusion or intravenous injection.

Stepwise search revealed the following references.

1. Gordon, M.A. et al.: Corneal Aspergillosis, *Am. Med. Assoc. Arch. Ophthalmol. 62*:758, 1959

2. Glassman, M.I. et al.: *Monosporium Apiospermum* Endophthalmitis, *Am. J. Ophthalmol. 76*:821, 1973

3. Ross, H.W. and Laibson, P.R.: Keratomycosis, *Am. J. Ophthalmol. 74*:438, 1972

4. Rosen, R. and Friedman, A.H.: Successfully Treated Postoperative *Candida Parakrusei* Endophthalmitis, *Am. J. Ophthalmol. 76*:574, 1973

5. Mangiaracine, A.B. and Liebman, S.D.: Fungus Keratitis (*Aspergillus fumigatus*), *Am. Med. Assoc. Arch. Ophthalmol. 58*:695, 1957

6. Havener, W. (Ed.): *Ocular Pharmacology,* 2nd edition, C.V. Mosby Company, St. Louis, Mo., pp. 481–482

7. Jones, D.B. et al.: *Fusarium solani* Keratitis Treated with Natamycin (Pimaricin®), *Arch. Ophthalmol. 88*:147, 1972

8. Blacow, N.W. (Ed.): *Martindale: The Extra Pharmacopoeia,* 26th Edition, The Pharmaceutical Press, London, England

9. *American Hospital Formulary Service,* American Society of Hospital Pharmacists (8:12.04)

Step IV. Response

Intraocular (topical) nystatin and amphotericin B have been successfully used in ocular fungal infections (keratomycosis, endophthalmitis).[1-5] Neither drug penetrates the eye satisfactorily by any other route than direct intraocular injection.[6]

Amphotericin B (Fungizone®) is almost insoluble in water. An ophthalmic solution, however, can be prepared from the base powder used for IV infusion. One vial contains 50 mg amphotericin B and about 41 mg sodium deoxycholate buffered with 25 mg sodium phosphate. The sodium deoxycholate complex increases the solubility of amphotericin B in water as a colloid. A 4 mg/ml suspension in sterile water has a pH of about 7.5.[7] The solution is prepared by adding sterile distilled water or 5 percent dextrose in water to produce the required concentration.[6,7] Saline must be avoided as it will precipitate the drug. Most studies have used concentrations of 1–5 mg/ml. Glassman et al.[2] recommend using 2.5–10 mg/ml in sterile water or 5 percent dextrose. Amphotericin B drops have been used as frequently as every fifteen minutes.

Nystatin (Mycostatin®) is also very insoluble in water. A 3 percent suspension in water has a pH of 6.5–8.0. A fine suspension may be prepared (25,000–100,000 units/ml) by adding normal saline to the Mycostatin® crystalline powder ("for laboratory use only").[1,2] If possible, the solution should be buffered to a pH of 7.0.[2] Alternately, up to 200,000 units may be dissolved in 1 ml of the special diluent provided by Squibb, which can then be added to isotonic saline or water to produce a fine suspension.[6] One other method has been described by Mangiaracine and Liebman.[5] Nystatin powder (500,000 units) is ground up and suspended in 10 ml of the following vehicle: sodium chloride 1.2 g, chlorobutanol 0.5 g, H_2O qs to 100 ml. This produces a 50,000 unit/ml suspension. The concentrations used vary from 25,000–100,000 units/ml. A suspension of 3000 units/ml (one drop instilled every $\frac{1}{2}$–1 hour) has been used successfully in keratomycosis.[3]

Both solutions are sensitive to light and heat and are inactivated in acidic or basic solutions. Both must be refrigerated. Amphotericin B solutions are stable for 24 hours at room temperature and for 7 days when stored at 4 °C (39 °F). Nystatin suspensions in water may be stable for up to one week at room temperature; refrigerated suspensions retain 90 percent of their original potency after refrigerated storage for 2 weeks.[6,8,9]

IX. Poisoning

What is in Tri-Aqua® (9/11/74)

Step I. Classification

1. Request. Drug identification (poisoning)

2. Requestor. Pharmacist

Comment. Although this appears at the outset to be a straight—forward identification question, it is rapidly changed by obtaining the appropriate background information.

Step II. Background Information

1. Patient Data. A $1\frac{1}{2}$-year-old boy (20 lb) has ingested approximately 20 Tri-Aqua® tablets.

2. Tri-Aqua® is an over-the-counter diuretic product, also sold by mail-order.

3. History. He was admitted Saturday night (9/8/74) in convulsions. Other symptoms were "clamping of jaws," pinpoint pupils and fluctuating periods of lethargy and extreme restlessness.

4. *Medication Data.* Phenobarbital injections (2 mg/kg) IM were given to control the seizures. IV fluids were started. Today he is extremely lethargic.

Comment. For all suspected ingestions, the following information must be obtained:

1. age, sex and weight of the victim;
2. name of the product (generic, brand name, chemical name), or description if unknown;
3. amount ingested, or an approximation;
4. method of exposure (oral, topical, inhalation). If not orally, elicit the amount and time of exposure;
5. time of exposure or ingestion, time of discovery, and beginning of treatment;
6. other disease states which may complicate symptoms or treatment (e.g., epilepsy, diabetes);
7. symptoms observed and treatment to date; and
8. other drugs the patient is receiving.

With this data, the poisoning can be placed into proper perspective and treatment based upon reliable information instituted. *Never* recommend therapy until all available background information has been elicited.

Obviously, not all this data can be obtained for every poisoning call, but an attempt to elicit as much data as possible will assist the pharmacist in searching for the product in question and in providing more accurate and useful information regarding the potential toxicity and treatment.

This particular call occurred "after the fact," that is, all expected symptoms had presented. At this point, a search to determine the consequences of Tri-Aqua® ingestion and any other treatment recommendations should be investigated.

Step III. Systematic Search

Comment. Useful references for poisoning calls are presented in Chapter 4. The most current and useful poison information source at present is the *POISINDEX*® system (see Chapter 4). Approximately 95 percent of all poison calls can be adequately handled with this system. If the *POISINDEX*® system is not available, then textbooks and other literature sources must be used.

The most useful texts at present are:

1. Gleason, et al.: *Clinical Toxicology of Commercial Products*
2. Dreisbach: *Handbook of Poisoning*
3. Deichman and Gerard: *Toxicology of Drugs and Chemicals*
4. Arena: *Poisoning: Toxicology—Symptoms—Treatments*

If the product cannot be identified from these sources, then the references used for drug identification questions (Chapter 4) should be consulted for ingredients. Then, if the identified product is not listed in these textbooks or if there is insufficient data, the manufacturer of the product should be contacted. Manufacturers are usually very helpful in supplying toxicological data regarding their products, especially during an acute ingestion, and most will accept collect calls from poison control centers. All drug information centers should attempt to maintain extensive toxicology files from all major manufacturers; many companies supply case histories of ingestions of their products and their treatment, which are not published in the literature.

A *TOXLINE* search and literature search may prove useful, if there is sufficient time. The most useful secondary literature sources for poisoning are:

1. *de Haen Drugs in Use;*
2. *InPharma;*
3. *Iowa Drug Information System;*

For the case presented here, the *POISINDEX®* system was not available. Tri-Aqua® was identified by calling the manufacturer, since it was not listed in the available identification reference sources. Then, toxicity and treatment were obtained by consulting two reference sources and using one article from the *Iowa System.* However, all of this data, as well as specific treatment, could have been located rapidly with the *POISINDEX®* system, which is highly useful for poison calls, as well as for other types of information (drug identification or availability, adverse drug reaction questions).

Stepwise search revealed the following references. ·

1. Personal Communications. Pfeiffer Lab., St. Louis, MO
2. Arena, J.: *Poisoning: Toxicology, Symptoms, Treatments* 3rd. Ed., Charles C Thomas, Springfield, Illinois, 1974
3. Gleason, M.N. et al.: *Clinical Toxicology of Commercial Products,* 3rd ed., Williams and Wilkins Co., Baltimore, 1969
4. Peters, J.M.: Factors affecting Caffeine Toxicity, *J. Clin. Pharmacol.* 1:131–140, 1967

Step IV. Response

Comment. Very seldom is it necessary to "write-up" answers to poisoning calls. Verbal responses are sufficient and the time factor limits the usefulness of writing-up the response. However, if documentation is required, the *POISINDEX®* system managements are usually all that are necessary, and these can be sent to the inquirer with the use of a viewer or printer.

With cases involving *chronic* poisoning, however, a written response is helpful, since the urgency of the response is not always immediate.

An example of a written response is presented here in order to enable the student to understand what a verbal response should consist of.

Tri-Aqua® is a weak diuretic consisting of bucher grass, caffeine (100 mg/tablet), zea, uva ursi and triticium.[1] The only toxic ingredient is caffeine alkaloid (100 mg/tablet). The lethal dose of caffeine is estimated to be 10 g in a 70 kg adult.[2] Assuming this child weighed approximately 10 kg, a lethal dose would be considered to be about 1.4 g. On the basis of the ingestion of 20 tablets, the child could have consumed 2 g of caffeine. However, fatal poisonings from caffeine are rare; we are aware of only 3 fatalities. The lowest dose resulting in death was 3.2 g (57 mg/kg) given IV.[3] In addition, sensitivity to caffeine appears to increase with age; infants and children are less sensitive to the toxic effects of caffeine than adults.[4]

The symptoms of caffeine overdose parallel somewhat the symptoms exhibited by this patient. They include restlessness, excitement, confusion, tremors, tachycardia, diarrhea, or irritability (which may alternate with drowsiness or lethargy) and rapid pulse. Nausea and emesis appear early and a bloody, syrup-like vomitus is eventually seen. These symptoms are followed by tremors, tonic extensor spasm interrupted by clonic convulsions, apathy, stupor and coma.[3] Absorption from the GI tract is unpredictable and there may be a long period between ingestion and the appearance of toxicity.

Treatment at this point should be supportive and symptomatic; parenteral fluids and electrolytes for dehydration and support of respiratory and cardiovascular function. Patients with convulsions from caffeine have recovered without treatment. The agent of choice for further seizures is diazepam (Valium®) 0.1 mg/kg IV. Further fluid replacement should be based on the patient's 24-hour urinary output.

What symptoms can be expected from chewing leaves of the plant Dumb Cane? (6/21/74)

Step I. Classification

1. *Request.* Poisoning
2. *Requestor.* Physician (pediatrician)

Step II. Background Information

1. *Patient Data.* An 8-month-old girl has chewed part of a leaf of Dumb Cane. She did not swallow any of the plant. Symptoms 10 minutes later included intense irritation and salivation.

Step III. Systematic Search

Comment. The references of choice for plant poisoning are the *POISINDEX®* system and the textbooks and articles listed in Chapter 4.

The most valuable textbooks are:

1. Lampe: *Plant Toxicity and Dermatitis*
2. Kingsbury: *Poisonous Plants of the United States and Canada*
3. Hardin: *Human Poisoning from Native and Cultivated Plants*
4. Ellis: *Dangerous Plants, Snakes, Arthropods and Marine Life—Toxicity and Treatment*

Several articles are also available which provide toxicology data on poisonous plants; one of the better references is an article by Arena entitled "The Perils in Plants" and published in *Emergency Medicine,* February, 1974.

A search of the literature (i.e., *Iowa System*) may also reveal case reports of plant poisoning, which are useful.

If a plant is *not* found in textbooks or other references, the chances are that it is not toxic. Emesis with ipecac is recommended for most plant ingestions, and is the treatment of choice when the offending plant cannot be located in reference sources.

Stepwise search revealed the following references.

1. Lampe, K.F. and Fagerstrom, R.: *Plant Toxicity and Dermatitis,* Williams and Wilkins Co., Baltimore, 1968, p. 12–13
2. Pohl, R.W.: Poisoning by Dieffenbachia, *J. Am. Med. Assoc. 117*:812, 1961
3. Drach, G. and Maloney, W.H.: Toxicity of the Common Houseplant Dieffenbachia. Report of a Case, *J. Am. Med. Assoc. 184*:1047–1048, 1963

Step IV. Response

Dieffenbachia spp. (Dumb Cane) are plants belonging to the family *Araceae.* They are chiefly gastroenteric irritants. After chewing, an intense burning sensation and increased salivation occurs, the speech may become thick and loss of voice has been reported to occur (hence the name, Dumb Cane). Severe edema of the buccal mucosa, tongue, palate and face may appear, which leads to dysphagia or a complete inability to swallow.[1] In some instances, contact may not produce immediate irritation.

Ingestion of the plant has only been reported rarely. If ingested, edema of the pharynx may be anticipated, together with serious gastroenteritis.[2]

Contact with the sap will produce dermatitis in susceptible individuals. Calcium oxalate is the main toxic ingredient, but renal injury or symptoms of tetany have not been reported. Since none of the plant was swallowed by this patient, treatment consists of relieving the intense pain in the mouth with meperidine.[3] Aluminum and magnesium hydroxide suspension should be given (1 oz every 2 hours), rinsed around the mouth and swallowed, if tolerated. Intravenous administration of glucose and saline may be required. Corticosteroids may be helpful, but the use of antihistamines has been disappointing. A diet of liquids and pureed foods should be instituted on the second or third day and the diet should remain restricted until all symptoms have abated.[1]

The edema should lessen in about 4 days and become minimal in about 12. The pain may be severe for up to 8 days. Superficial necrosis on the tongue and buccal mucosa may be expected.[1]

Can chronic exposure to carbon monoxide lead to parkinsonism? (11/20/75)

Step I. Classification

1. *Request.* Poisoning (chronic)
2. *Requestor.* Physician

Step II. Background Information

1. Two patients at a local smelting plant have been exposed to carbon monoxide fumes for about 20 years. Carbon disulfide vapors are also present (p.p.m. not disclosed).
2. One patient has developed a definite parkinsonism tremor in the past 2 years and is currently receiving levodopa.
3. The other patient has recently developed a fine tremor of an undefined nature (possible essential tremor). The use of propranolol has been considered.
4. Both patients have filed law suits against the plant, suggesting that dangerously high levels of carbon monoxide gas are the cause of their symptoms.

Comment. This is a typical question involving chronic toxicity or poisoning. The response was not of an urgent nature and was used in court. Thus, the pharmacist did a relatively thorough search of the literature and prepared a complete, written report.

Step III. Systematic Search

Comment. Toxicology textbooks and the *POISINDEX*® system are good starting points for chronic poisoning cases and often cite primary references which can be used to formulate the response. If nothing is found in these references, then the use of secondary literature sources is necessary. The sources used are the same as for adverse reaction questions (see Chapter 4).

In this particular instance, no cases of parkinsonism secondary to CO exposure had been reported in the previous 10 years.

However, several texts and articles did mention that this disease had been previously reported to result from CO exposure, but no specific details were given. Thus, a search, via *Index Medicus*, was instituted of the literature prior to 1964. This revealed several articles, which in turn led to more articles from their bibliography. In addition, one textbook (*Industrial Toxicology*, Hamilton and Hardy) presented a good review of the condition, as well as some primary references.

Stepwise search revealed the following references.

1. Sax, N.: *Dangerous Properties of Industrial Materials*, 4th Ed, Van Nostrand Reinhold Company, New York, 1975, pp. 520–521

2. Grinker, R.: Parkinsonism Following Carbon Monoxide Poisoning, *J. Nerv. Ment. Dis.* 64:18, 1926

3. Raskin, N. and Mullaney, O.: The Mental and Neurological Sequelae of Carbon Monoxide Asphyxia in a Case Observed for Fifteen Years, *J. Nerv. Ment. Dis.* 92:640, 1940

4. Sanger, E. and Gilliland, W.: Severe Carbon Monoxide Poisoning with Prolonged Coma, *J. Am. Med. Assoc.*: Jan 27, 1940

5. Gilbert, G. and Glaser, G.: Neurologic Manifestations of Chronic Carbon Monoxide Poisoning, *N. Engl. J. Med.* 261:1217, 1959

6. Solomon, A.: Acalculia, Other Agnosias and Multiple Neuritis Following Carbon Monoxide Poisoning, *Med. Clin. North Am.*:531, 1932

7. Shillito, F. et al.: The Problem of Nervous and Mental Sequelae in Carbon Monoxide Poisoning, *J. Am. Med. Assoc.* 106:669, 1936

8. Beck, H.: Slow Carbon Monoxide Asphyxiation, *J. Am. Med. Assoc.*, 107:1025, 1936

9. Jackson, R. et al.: Case of Carbon Monoxide Poisoning with Complications, *Br. Med. J.* 2:1130, 1959

10. Papavasiliou, P. et al.: Levodopa in Parkinsonism: Potentiation of Central Effects with a Peripheral Inhibitor, *N. Engl. J. Med.* 285:8, 1972

11. Rowan, T. and Coleman, F.: Carbon Monoxide Poisoning, *J. For. Sci.* 7:103, 1962

12. Hamilton and Hardy: *Industrial Toxicology,* pp. 239–258

Step IV. Response

Comment. In this case, the physician requested a thorough summary of the literature in a logical format. Therefore, the response presented a brief summary of each case in the literature, with appropriate conclusions based on the findings. Thus, on occasion, the *format of the response* should be based upon the specific needs of the requestor. At all times, however, the response should be *tailored* to the needs of the requestor; that is, usable information should be presented, based upon careful evaluation of background data and findings in literature.

A syndrome of parkinsonism has been described following acute and chronic exposure to carbon monoxide, although case reports of this effect are almost nonexistent in the literature. There have been absolutely no cases of this nature recorded in the last 10 years.

Carbon disulfide is also formed and liberated in the furnaces at the smelting plant and chronic exposure to this agent can also result in CNS damage.[1] In chronic poisoning with carbon disulfide, the picture is one of involvement of the CNS, with neuritis and disturbance of vision being the most common early changes. Often there is pain in the limbs and these symptoms are followed by muscular weakness and wasting. Mental symptoms may vary from simple excitation or depression and irritability in mild cases, to mental deterioration, parkinsonian paralysis and even insanity. These changes are accompanied by insomnia, loss of memory and personality changes.[1]

The following is a review of the literature describing parkinsonian reactions following CO exposure.

Grinker[2] describes a case of what he terms "myelinopathy" following acute carbon monoxide poisoning which resulted in parkinsonism in a 58-year-old female. Whether or not this case presented as true parkinsonism is debatable, as there were no involuntary tremors or hyperkinesias but only pure rigidity. These symptoms occurred about one month after acute exposure.

Raskin and Mullaney[3] described parkinsonism as a sequelae to carbon monoxide asphyxia in a 33-year-old female. Coarse, irregular tremors of the outstretched hands developed about 6 years after her exposure to carbon monoxide. She also suffered from a tremor of the palate and lips which gradually worsened and resulted in marked chattering of her teeth. These symptoms progressed and the patient died of bronchopneumonia 15 years following the acute exposure. The anatomical findings consisted of a large bilateral, symmetrical necrosis of globus pallidus and small glial scars throughout the cortex, with the corresponding areas of demyelination, milk vascular and neuronal changes.

Sanger et al.[4] described a parkinsonian syndrome in a 27-year-old male about 3 weeks after 6 hours of exposure to carbon monoxide. The patient remained in varying degrees of coma for about 12 days. Parkinsonism was evident on the 16th day after exposure to CO and persisted for over a month, disappearing gradually.

Gilbert and Glaser[5] imply that it is difficult to distinguish chronic intoxication with CO as compared to repeated acute exposures. They describe a case of chronic CO poisoning of several years duration in a 50-year-old male. Symptoms during and after 4 years of exposure to CO gas (in a garage) consisted of a fine, rapid tremor of the fingers and broad-based gait. The tremors seemed to increase in frequency over the 4-year period. Whether or not these are parkinsonian symptoms is debatable; however, the patient was not responding to anticonvulsant drugs.

Solomon[6] describes 2 cases of carbon monoxide exposure

resulting in almost unquestionable parkinsonism. Both patients exhibited classic parkinsonian symptoms several days after the exposure. These symptoms have persisted in one patient.

Shillito et al.[7] examined the clinical characteristics of the nervous sequelae following carbon monoxide asphyxia in 43 patients. All cases showed a fairly high incidence of neurologic changes, which appeared soon after the intoxication along with mental manifestations. Several patients exhibited well advanced parkinsonism, with increased reflexes, slow movement, lack of coordination, fixed facies and scanning speech. Six patients suffered permanent neurologic sequelae. Five of these patients have permanent effects of parkinsonism and one simply had increased reflexes.

Beck[8] states that carbon monoxide anoxemia may unquestionably produce a parkinsonian syndrome, which so frequently accompanies other forms of encephalitis, as well as any of the many other encephalitic symptoms, as the pathology is essentially the same as for epidemic encephalitis.

Jackson et al.[9] indicate that parkinsonism is a common sequelae to carbon monoxide poisoning, since the basal ganglia are considered a locus minoris resistentiae to carbon monoxide.

Papavasiliou et al.[10] report the results of levodopa and carbidopa in several patients with parkinsonism, one being a child with parkinsonism secondary to carbon monoxide poisoning.

Excellent review articles with discussions of parkinsonism as a neurological sequelae from acute and chronic carbon monoxide poisoning have been prepared by Rowan and Coleman[11] and Hamilton and Hardy.[12]

Conclusion. It is evident from these reports that symptoms of parkinsonism can result from single acute exposures to carbon monoxide, or repeated acute insults over a long period of time. These symptoms are apparently due to damage of the basal ganglion. Carbon disulfide should also be considered as a possible etiologic agent in these patients. Recovery is not always complete and the patient should obviously be removed from further carbon monoxide insults.

Index